10:00 7th
s.
D0887437

Learning Activities for Life Span Motor Development
Third Edition

Kathleen M. Haywood, PhD
Nancy Getchell, PhD
University of Missouri–St. Louis

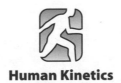

Human Kinetics

Library of Congress Cataloging-in-Publication Data

Haywood, Kathleen.
    Learning activities for life span motor development third edition / Kathleen M.
Haywood, Nancy Getchell.
        p. cm.
    Includes bibliogrphical references.
    ISBN 0-7360-4019-6
    1. Motor ability in children--Laboratory manuals. 2. Motor ability--Laboratory
manuals. I. Getchell, Nancy, 1963- II. Haywood, Kathleen. Life span motor
development. 3rd ed. III. Title.

RJ133 .H339 2001
612.7'6--dc21

                                                                        2001024713

ISBN: 0-7360-4019-6

Copyright © 2001 by Kathleen M. Haywood and Nancy Getchell
Copyright © 1993, 1988 by Kathleen M. Haywood

All rights reserved. Except for use in a review, the reproduction or utilization of this work in any form or by any electronic, mechanical, or other means, now known or hereafter invented, including xerography, photocopying, and recording, and in any information storage and retrieval system, is forbidden without the written permission of the publisher.

Notice: Permission to reproduce the following material is granted to instructors and agencies who have purchased *Learning Activities for Life Span Motor Development Third Edition:* pages 7, 9, 13, 16–18, 24, 30, 33, 37, 40, 43, 49, 51, 54–55, 70–71, 74–75, 78, 85, 91, 97, 107–108, 113–114, 120, 123–124, 129, 134, 137–140, 145, 149–150, 153, 157, 160, 164–165, 170, 176, 179, 197, 201, 206. The reproduction of other parts of this book is expressly forbidden by the above copyright notice. Persons or agencies who have not purchased *Learning Activities for Life Span Motor Development Third Edition* may not reproduce any material.

This book is a revised edition of *Laboratory Activities for Life Span Motor Development,* second edition, published in 1993 by Human Kinetics.

Acquisitions Editor: Judy Patterson Wright, PhD; **Developmental Editor:** Melissa Feld; **Assistant Editor:** Susan C. Hagan; **Copyeditor:** Joyce Sexton; **Proofreader:** Myla Smith; **Permission Manager:** Dalene Reeder; **Graphic Designer:** Robert Reuther; **Graphic Artist:** Dawn Sills; **Photo Manager:** Clark Brooks; **Cover Designer:** Keith Blomberg; **Photographers (cover):** Clark Brooks and Tom Roberts; **Photographer (interior):** Tom Roberts, unless otherwise noted. Photos on pages 46–48, 83, 88, 95, 102, 111, 131, and 224 provided by the authors; **Art Manager:** Craig Newsom; **Illustrator:** Mic Greenberg; **Printer:** Versa Press

Printed in the United States of America

10 9 8 7 6 5 4 3 2 1

Human Kinetics
Web site: www.humankinetics.com

United States: Human Kinetics
P.O. Box 5076
Champaign, IL 61825-5076
800-747-4457
e-mail: humank@hkusa.com

Canada: Human Kinetics
475 Devonshire Road Unit 100
Windsor, ON N8Y 2L5
800-465-7301 (in Canada only)
e-mail: orders@hkcanada.com

Europe: Human Kinetics
Units C2/C3 Wira Business Park
West Park Ring Road
Leeds LS16 6EB, United Kingdom
+44 (0) 113 278 1708
e-mail: hk@hkeurope.com

Australia: Human Kinetics
57A Price Avenue
Lower Mitcham, South Australia 5062
08 8277 1555
e-mail: liahka@senet.com.au

New Zealand: Human Kinetics
P.O. Box 105-231, Auckland Central
09-523-3462
e-mail: hkp@ihug.co.nz

Contents

CONTENTS

Preface

In all of the *Life Span Motor Development* resources, we stress that motor development is more than just a college course. It represents the movement aspect of our lives as we proceed through the life span. For some people, it is their very careers. It also is a perspective, a way of looking at events in life in the context of age-related change. You can just "read about" and "learn about" motor development. Better, though, is for you to experience it. Numerous opportunities exist for engaging motor development topics by observing, participating, and exchanging ideas with others. The goal of *Learning Activities for Life Span Motor Development* is to suggest and provide for some of those experiences. There might be no other college course as well suited to experiential activities as one in motor development!

Indeed, the very model used in the *Life Span Motor Development* text reminds us that movement arises as the interaction among an individual, the task that the individual undertakes, and the environment in which the individual exists. Considering the change in an individual without considering that person's context is limiting. A more complete understanding and appreciation of how movement changes over the life span is achieved when movement is considered, studied, observed, and experienced in its environmental context. The purpose of this learning activities guide is to provide you with activities that promote understanding of the most important concepts discussed in the textbook. Many of the activities suggested here allow for that very experience in a movement setting.

Studying motor development across the life span can seem like a daunting task, considering the different constraints (individual, environmental, task) that affect movement behavior. For that reason, we have expanded the laboratory activities guide that accompanied *Life Span Motor Development*, second edition, into a learning activities guide for the third edition. The activities suggested in this guide are of various types. Some involve direct observations of individuals at various points in the life span with follow-up analysis and discussion. Others involve watching individuals in video clips on your CD-ROM. Still others involve analyzing data provided in this text. So, there are various ways to engage and explore the many aspects of motor development.

The study of motor development should be enjoyable and engaging as well as beneficial. In short, you have been, are, and will continue to be developing motorically! We hope you find *Learning Activities for Life Span Motor Development Third Edition* a useful, challenging, and, above all, interesting way to learn about motor development. Enjoy the exploration of motor development on both a personal and a professional level.

How to Use the CD-ROM

On the CD-ROM included with this text, you will find video presentations to be used with exercises in chapters 1, 5, 6, 7, 8, and 9. The individuals in the video clips on your CD-ROM should be very much like those you might observe in the role of teacher, coach, or therapist. They were not chosen as "special" models for the CD-ROM and we did not ask them to perform in any special way or look like someone in particular. Also, we tried to film them in realistic settings rather than in a research laboratory. Since they are "real" performers, you might find that some of them do not fit clearly into a developmental level or do not look exactly like the drawings in your text. This is exactly what you find in realistic settings! Sometimes placing an individual into a developmental level involves watching several times over and making a best judgment. We recall an expert colleague, struggling over whether a child should be placed into developmental level 2 or developmental level 3, saying, "this child is exactly in developmental level 2.5!" Always keep in mind that you can make note of the unique characteristics demonstrated by an individual, even while making your best judgment on where they should be placed in the developmental sequence of movement characteristics.

While we intend for the video clips to show "real" performers, they are indeed video clips and you should feel free to take advantage of this. Watch them in slow motion by dragging the scrubber bar from left to right, stop the action in critical places, or change the rate of speed so that you can see the critical positions and relationships of the limbs and trunk. This is actually the preferred way to categorize performers into developmental levels until you have the experience to do it "live" and in real time!

What Is on the CD?

The clips in chapter 1 are intended to get you started observing. You will rank individuals on a throwing task from least to most advanced. In chapter 5, we provide video clips that show several different points of development in infancy and toddlerhood; we ask you to put the clips into a developmental order. In chapter 6, we provide video clips of locomotor, ballistic, and manipulative skills. The chapter is divided into five folders: standing long jump, hopping, overarm throw, kicking, and catching. You will rank the clips in chapter 6 from least to most developmentally advanced using the principles of motion and stability as a guide.

For chapters 7, 8, and 9, more than one learning activity in the chapter uses video clips, so you will have to select the folder labeled for the skill you are observing, such as throwing or striking. We have further subdivided the video clips in chapters 7, 8, and 9 into two folders. We have called the first folder "Set A: Guided Practice." Each Set A: Guided Practice folder provides two video clips with scripts that guide you through the observation plans to the appropriate category of each developmental sequence. These interactive video clips allow you to practice using the observation plan and provide the correct answer. The second folder within each skill is called "Set B: Assessment Practice." These video clips do not have scripts. You will need to work through the observation plan on your own to categorize the developmental sequence for each individual. Your instructor may assign these clips for tests, homework assignments, or in conjunction with a learning activity. Instructors will find our categorizations of the developmental sequences for chapters 1, 5, and 6 and the Set B: Assessment Practice video clips in chapters 7, 8, and 9 in the Instructor Guide.

Installing the CD-ROM and Getting Started

To begin, you need to follow the installation and getting started procedures included on the inside back cover. Once you have opened the program, click on "Begin." You will then be able to click on the appropriate chapter number; you can also navigate by using the directory to the left of the main screen. Once you have opened a folder containing the video clips, you will see the various clips that are available, labeled "Example 1," "Example 2," and so on. Choose the one you want, and you are set to observe!

Viewing the Video Clips

On the CD-ROM we have included a help file that provides information on how to use and navigate through the CD. Please open the help file for complete information on using the CD-ROM. Below we have provided tips on how to take advantage of the CD-ROM features.

The Directory

Once you get past the main title screen of the CD-ROM, a directory will appear to the left of the video screen. You can use the directory to navigate through the CD-ROM. You can move it to a different position on your desktop by clicking on the main title bar and dragging it to a new location. You can also adjust the size of the directory by clicking and dragging on a corner of the directory until you reach the desired size. After you have moved the directory, you can easily put it back in its original position by clicking on Options and then Dock Directory.

Moving from Clip to Clip

There are two ways to move from one clip to another. First, you may simply click on each example in the directory that you want to view. Second, on the main video screen there are two red arrows to the left and right of the video. Clicking on the arrow to the left moves you back one clip and clicking on the arrow to the right moves you forward one clip. However, when you are in the Set A: Guided Practice clips, you will move through the entire observation plan before you can move on to the next clip, unless you click "Exit Test."

Adjusting the Speed of the Clips

You can watch at regular speed by clicking on the "play" arrow or at slow speed by dragging the cursor below the picture. You can also adjust the rate of speed by moving the bar to the right of the main video screen up and down.

The Loop Button

To view the video clip continuously, click on the loop button located at the bottom right corner of the video screen. This allows the clip to repeat until you uncheck the button. While you are working through the observation plans, you may find it helpful to loop the clip as you answer the questions.

Answering the Set A Questions

As mentioned previously, Set A clips are designed to take you through the process of developmental sequence categorization by asking questions from the appropriate observation plan. You will be given two choices for each question. Once you make your selection, click on Continue to find out if you answered the question correctly. Once you have answered the question correctly you will be moved on to the next question.

PART I

Introduction to Motor Development

CHAPTER 1

Fundamental Concepts

It is much easier to study an area when we can see many ties to our own lives and many issues relevant to our chosen careers. Motor development is certainly an area of study that we can all identify with. We can find many developmental topics and issues as we read newspapers and news magazines, listen to news radio, and watch television news and feature-story programs. All of us are aging, and all of us have family members and friends who are aging (remember, infants begin aging as soon as they are born!). So issues of development are all around us, including those that involve our physical growth and aging and our ability to move in order to engage in activities of daily living, as well as recreation.

Although developmental issues can be interesting to us all, development in general, as well as motor development in particular, is a formal area of study. As such it entails specific terminology and common methods of acquiring information and examining issues. Often, the scientific method is applied to developmental research questions. Motor development terminology and method of study need not be mysterious. We all simply need to become familiar with how motor developmentalists go about their business. Some of the learning activities in this chapter are designed to familiarize you with the tools developmentalists use to study motor development. Other activities are designed to make you more comfortable with the research process. They will provide you with the building blocks for the subsequent chapters. So, students of motor development need to learn facts about motor development and the tools and methods of inquiry used in the field.

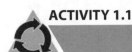

ACTIVITY 1.1

Observation As a Tool of Inquiry

Purpose: To gain experience observing movement.

As we just acknowledged, students of motor development need to learn both facts and tools of inquiry in motor development. One of the tools of inquiry in motor development is observation. In fact, developmentalists during the 20th century gained a reputation for being keen, careful, and methodical observers of human behavior. This is particularly true with regard to the observation of motor skills. In the 1920s and 1930s, developmentalists put more emphasis on thorough observation of a few individuals than on observation of large numbers of individuals. Even so, observations of the motor milestone skills in that era were so accurate that we are able to use much of the information today. Sharp observation skills never go out of date!

Moreover, scientists are not the only ones who use observation when it comes to the field of motor development. Teachers, coaches, and therapists must be every bit as skilled in the use of observation. Throughout this text we will put much emphasis on environments and tasks that interact with growing and aging individuals to give rise to movement. Practitioners typically do not change the growing and aging processes, but they frequently adapt environments and tasks for those with whom they work. These adaptations can allow children to enjoy certain movement tasks, can allow individuals with disabilities to live independently, can promote the recovery of those who have sustained injuries, can keep seniors moving, and so on! Effective adaptations usually follow accurate observation of the interactions among individuals, environments, and tasks and careful analysis of the resulting movements.

Of course, students of motor development need to know *what* to observe as well as *how* to observe. This takes time. Of course, you are just beginning! Yet you might know more than you would think, or you might be able to derive more from reflections of your observations than you would guess. As a way to get warmed up to observation as a tool of inquiry in motor development, in this activity you will observe some movers. You will make some initial judgments about what you observe. As you learn more about motor development, you will have the opportunity later to reconsider your judgments.

Instructions

1. On your CD-ROM, in the Chapter 1 folder, you will see four files named "Example 1" through "Example 4." Each shows an individual throwing overhand, and each of the individuals is at a different developmental level. Watch each movie. You can watch at regular speed by clicking on the "play" arrow, watch at slow speed by dragging the cursor below the video, or adjust the rate of speed by moving the bar to the left of the video up or down. Watch the clips as many times as you like.

2. Decide which of the four throwers is the most developmentally advanced. Now decide which among the remaining three is the most advanced, and then which of the remaining two is more advanced. The one left is the thrower you believe is the least developmentally advanced. Record your decisions from most to least advanced in the box on the next page.

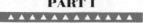
Most advanced			Least advanced
_____	_____	_____	_____

Questions

1. What types of information did you use to make your decisions: body position, movements, speed of movement, body size, apparent age, and so on?
2. What did you decide were the characteristics of a developmentally advanced throw? That is, what information did you ultimately use in making your decisions?
3. What made your decisions easy? What made them difficult? Why?

In chapter 8 we will discuss the characteristics of developmentally advanced throws, as well as the characteristics of many other fundamental motor skills. You can then review your decisions to see how well you did.

 ACTIVITY 1.2

Formulating Developmental Research Questions

Purpose: To examine developmental research questions and see what distinguishes them from other research questions.

Few of us think of ourselves as researchers, yet we all periodically ask ourselves about relationships in our world. You might ask yourself what the relationship is between that squeaking noise and the stopping ability of your car when you apply the brakes, or the relationship between the time you spent studying and the grade you earned on your last exam.

Researchers ask questions about relationships just as we all do, but they follow up by answering the question through systematic and controlled observations. In that way they provide us all with new information—information that can cure us of disease or injury, lead to the development of devices that make life more convenient, or tell us which instructional methods are most effective.

Simple research questions involve two variables (things that can have multiple values or levels), but many researchers ask questions that involve three or more variables. For example, a research question might be: what is the relationship of height and weight to the distance one can jump vertically? The variables are height, weight, and distance jumped. Another research question might be: what is the relationship between auditory acuity and ability to detect high-frequency sounds among various age groups? The variables are auditory acuity, detection of high-frequency sound, and age.

Note that a research question does not state _what_ the relationship is. Rather, it is a _hypothesis_ that makes this type of statement. A research question simply addresses whether there is a relationship among height, weight, and vertical-jump distance or among whatever other variables one is studying. A hypothesis would state the possible direction of the relationship—for example, the shorter and heavier one is, the shorter one's vertical jump. There is not a "right" or "wrong" direction for a hypothesis. A researcher usually hypothesizes the direction that would be predicted from previous studies; but until the research is conducted we really do not know whether there is a relationship among the variables at all, and if there is, what the direction of that relationship is.

In your study of development, it is important to recognize which research topics concern developmental issues and which do not. Mary Ann Roberton (1988, p. 130) proposes using the following "test" to decide whether a question is or is not developmental. Ask these three questions:

1. Is the interest in what a behavior or status is like *now*, and why the behavior is the way it is?
2. Is the interest in what a behavior or status was like *before*, and why?
3. Is the interest in how this behavior or status is *going to change* in the future, and why?

We typically answer *yes* to the first question for any research question; but if we also answer *yes* to the second and third questions, then we know that the research topic is a developmental one. For example, suppose a researcher is interested in the relationship between depth perception and basketball shooting accuracy. If the researcher studies this relationship in one age group, the answers to the second and third questions are *no*. If, instead, the researcher is interested in the change in depth perception during adolescence and basketball shooting accuracy, the answers are *yes*, and we know that the research issue is a developmental one. Notice that in the developmental research question there are three variables, namely age, depth perception, and shooting accuracy.

In this learning activity you will form some research questions and then decide whether they are developmental questions or not. Your questions can take the following form: Is there a relationship between _____ and _____ ? The blanks are variables—things that can vary in value, level, or status. For example, age varies. People, animals, and objects can be of a specific age within a range of possible ages. Gender varies, too, although between just two possibilities, male and female. So, the levels or values of a variable can be numerical or categorical. Sometimes researchers group numerical values into categories. For example, the variable "reaction time" can be expressed as a number of milliseconds, or as a category representing numerical values, such as "slow," "moderate," or "fast."

Table 1.1 lists two sets of variables. Use these variables in your learning activities. You can see that all these items can vary in level, value, or status.

TABLE 1.1

Individual variables	Task variables
Height	Diameter of a ball
Leg length	Weight of a ball
Sitting height	Height of a net
Visual acuity	Width of a goal
Flexibility	Height of a keyboard table
Reaction time	Height of a kitchen countertop
Hand-eye coordination	Distance to a road sign
Age	
Physiological maturation	
Stage of development	

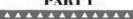
Instructions

1. Working just from the list of individual variables, choose two variables and formulate a research question in the format "Is there a relationship between _____ and _____ ?" Record your research question on record sheet 1.1.

2. Do this three additional times with pairs of different variables. Record your research questions on the record sheet.

3. Examine your four research questions. Apply the Roberton questions to test whether each of your questions is developmental or not, and state the results of your analysis on the record sheet.

4. If none of your questions is developmental, what is a variable that, if you had included it, would have made the question developmental? Formulate that research question and record it. If all of your questions are developmental, substitute a variable that would change the question so it is not developmental. Formulate this new question.

5. What are the variables from the list of individual variables, then, that often make a research question developmental? Why? Record the variables you have selected, and your rationale, on the record sheet.

6. Now formulate a research question using two individual variables and one task variable, including a variable that makes the question developmental. Again, record this research question.

7. Do this three additional times, formulating one more developmental question and two questions that are not developmental. Record these questions on the record sheet.

8. Select any two of your developmental research questions. Now you get to hypothesize the direction of the relationship between or among your variables. For example, "The older adults get, the poorer their auditory acuity and the harder it is for them to detect high-frequency sounds." Record your hypotheses on the record sheet.

Developmental Research Questions

Research questions with two individual variables	Is this a developmental research question?
1.	
2.	
3.	
4.	

Reformulated research question:_____

_____

The variables that make a research question developmental are:_____

_____

Your rationale:_____

_____

Research questions with two individual and one task variable
1. (Developmental)
2. (Developmental)
3. (Not developmental)
4. (Not developmental)

Hypothesis
1.
2.

From *Learning Activities for Life Span Motor Development Third Edition* by Kathleen Haywood and Nancy Getchell, 2001, Champaign, IL: Human Kinetics.

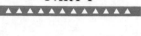
ACTIVITY 1.3

Designing a Developmental Research Study

Purpose: To understand how researchers design developmental research studies by designing two studies using research questions from activity 1.2.

In casually reading the results of a research study, we might not think about why a researcher conducted the study in a particular way. Then, we might overlook how the design of the study influences or delimits its results. Our understanding of motor development research can be more complete (and the process seem less mysterious) if we understand more about the process of designing research studies.

In this activity, you will design two research studies based on two of the developmental research questions you wrote in activity 1.2.

Instructions

1. Select a developmental research question from activity 1.2. Decide whether your study will be longitudinal, cross-sectional, or sequential. Record the chosen question and its type on record sheet 1.2.

2. Decide whom you will measure or observe, and enter this information on the record sheet. (Assume for now that you will measure or observe groups of individuals with a particular characteristic, e.g., individuals who are 8 years of age, rather than just an individual or two.)

3. Decide when you will measure them, and record this information on the record sheet.

4. Decide what you will measure or observe (what individual characteristic, behavior, etc.) and record it appropriately.

5. Consider all of your variables. Have you allowed for each of them to vary, that is, to have two or more levels or values? For example, if gender is one of your variables, have you included both males and females? If age is one of your variables, do you have two or more age groups or two or more ages of observation? If your answer is *no*, change your methods so that you can answer *yes*. A space on the record sheet is provided for such a change.

6. Notice that you as researcher control the levels of some variables, that is, you include both levels of gender or decide to observe 9-, 11-, and 13-year-olds. These are termed *independent variables*. Which one or two of your variables are independent? List the independent variable(s) on your record sheet.

7. Notice, too, that there are some variables you do not "set" by choosing their levels. Rather, you will observe the behavior of the subjects included in your study. These variables are labeled *dependent variables*, since (assuming they are indeed related to your independent variables) their value or level *depends* on the value or level of the independent variable(s) in your study. Which are your dependent variables? Record them appropriately.

8. Write a hypothesis for your research question, that is, a statement in which you speculate on the *direction* of any relationship between or among your variables, and enter it on the record sheet.

9. Repeat this process with another of your developmental research questions, making the appropriate entries on record sheet 1.2.

Designing a Developmental Research Study

First Question

Your research question and type of design: _____

_____

Whom you will observe: _____

When you will observe them: _____

What will you measure/observe? _____

Do your variables have two or more levels? If not, your change: _____

Independent variable(s): _____

Dependent variable(s): _____

Hypothesis: _____

_____

Second Question

Your research question and type of design: _____

_____

Whom you will observe: _____

When you will observe them: _____

What will you measure/observe? _____

Do your variables have two or more levels? If not, your change: _____

Independent variable(s): _____

Dependent variable(s): _____

Hypothesis: _____

_____

From *Learning Activities for Life Span Motor Development Third Edition* by Kathleen Haywood and Nancy Getchell, 2001, Champaign, IL: Human Kinetics.

Questions

1. If you actually conducted a study on one of these research questions, would you be able to say whether the results support your hypothesis or not? How?

2. What did you find easy or difficult about designing your studies? Why?

ACTIVITY 1.4

Graphing Developmental Data

Purpose: To gain proficiency in interpreting graphs of developmental data and presenting developmental information to others with a graph.

Researchers believe in the old saying that "a picture is worth a thousand words" just as much as any of us, the difference being that their "pictures" are graphs of the data they collect in research projects. Graphs can show trends over time at a glance—giving them a great advantage over a page full of numbers! Once you know how to read graphs, you will have a time-saving skill at your disposal; and once you know how to create them, you will have a powerful communication tool. Of course, graphing is an easy process today because there are so many computer software programs that do much of the work for us. Still, the software user must know how to direct the program to set up the graph. In this activity you gain experience setting up graphs, interpreting graphs, and graphing data, both by hand and with computer software. The following are some general principles.

1. Since development involves age-related change, most graphs of developmental data picture information over an age range. The convention in graphing is to make the horizontal axis the one for age or time.

2. Naturally, then, the vertical axis is used to plot the measurement of those in the study (the dependent variable). Typically, one kind of measurement is pictured per graph. While there can be exceptions, for now we will put just one measurement on a graph.

3. Graphs can picture individuals' measurements or group averages. If too many individuals or groups are graphed on one chart, the chart can become impossible to read. There is no "rule" as to how many individuals or groups can appear on one graph; the number often depends on the extent of overlap in the data.

In setting up the horizontal and vertical axes, consider the range of numbers to be plotted, and then bracket that range. For example, if you are plotting weights between 11 and 37 kg, make 10 kg the lowest point on the axis and 40 the highest. It often is tempting to choose larger, round numbers, say 0 and 50. This leaves blank spaces in your graph and forces the interesting data into a smaller area, making them difficult to see. Make short index lines on your graph for major reference points on that axis. For our weight example, index lines could be 15, 20, 25, 30, and 35.

More often than not, you will put lower numbers to the left on the horizontal axis and at the bottom on the vertical axis. The result is that the graphed line, or the bars in a bar graph, go up—the most natural direction for most developmental data. Of course not all measurements go "up" with advancing age, but it is still our preference to set up graphs of developmental data in this direction. Some measurements are scaled such that a lower number is better. A good example is the case of plotting the number of errors or incorrect responses. The fewer, the better! In this case, you probably want the larger numbers on

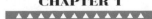

the bottom such that improved performance with the passage of time is a line going up. In reading graphs you should consider the axes and the type of measure being plotted before you interpret the meaning of lines going up and down, just to make sure that "up" represents "more" or "better."

If you have a variable in your study other than age and the measurement or observation (dependent variable), you can represent it in your graph by plotting one level of the variable with one line, the second level with a second line, the third level with a third line, and so on. It is helpful to use different types of lines or different colors. For example, you might graph the weight of boys from 6 to 10 years of age with a solid line and the weight of girls from 6 to 10 with a dashed line. Alternatively, you can use different symbols—say, an "x" or "o" or a triangle—for the different levels of the variable.

Instructions

1. Consider table 1.2. It contains the average (or mean) height in centimeters of a group of children for every year starting with their fourth birthdays and ending with their ninth (i.e., these are longitudinal data). Select your low and high values for each axis, and enter these values on the graph on record sheet 1.3 on p. 13. Now label some index lines on each axis. On your graph, place an "X" where the 4 on your age axis and 107 on your height axis intersect. Continue in this way until you have plotted each average height. Connect these data points to form a line.

2. Now, let us assume that you have just plotted average height for a group of North American children and that a friend in Australia sends you the average height measurements for a group of Australian children. These average heights are in table 1.3. Plot these averages on the same graph as before, using a small triangle for your data points and connecting them with a dashed line.

3. Consider table 1.4. It contains average scores in centimeters on the "sit-and-reach" flexibility test for four groups of boys: one group age 15, one group age 16, one group age 17, and one group age 18. It also contains average scores for four groups of girls: one group age 15, and so on (i.e., these are cross-sectional data). Type the data in table 1.4 into a software program designed for spreadsheets, such as Microsoft® Excel®.

4. Have the software program show your data on a line graph/chart (you may have to identify or highlight the data to be graphed). By generating a line graph/chart we are assuming that the various age groups represent the measurements we would have attained by measuring one group for 4 years. Print your graph and submit it with your record sheet.

5. Let us say that you suspect a strong cohort effect, such as the younger two groups' having a teacher who led daily stretching exercises. You decide that a bar graph would be more appropriate. Have the program plot a bar graph and print the graph. Submit it with your record sheet.

Questions

1. Examine the first line that you plotted on your graph. What does it tell you about height between 4 and 9 years of age in this group of children? According to this graph, does height increase the same amount every year? If not, what would the graph have to look like for height to increase the same amount every year?

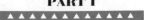
2. What does the graph tell you about the growth in height of the Australian children? Compare the growth in height of North American and Australian children as shown by this graph (remember, these are not real data).

3. What does the graph that you generated with computer software tell you about age-related trends in flexibility? About these trends in boys versus girls?

4. What did you find easier about doing the graph by computer compared to doing the graph by hand? What was more difficult?

TABLE 1.2

Age	4	5	6	7	8	9
Height (cm)	107	114	122	127	131	137

TABLE 1.3

Age	4	5	6	7	8	9
Height (cm)	103	110	118	126	133	137

TABLE 1.4

Age (years)	15	16	17	18
Boys (cm)	34.3	35.8	36.6	36.6
Girls (cm)	39.1	41.9	40.6	40.1

Graphing Developmental Data

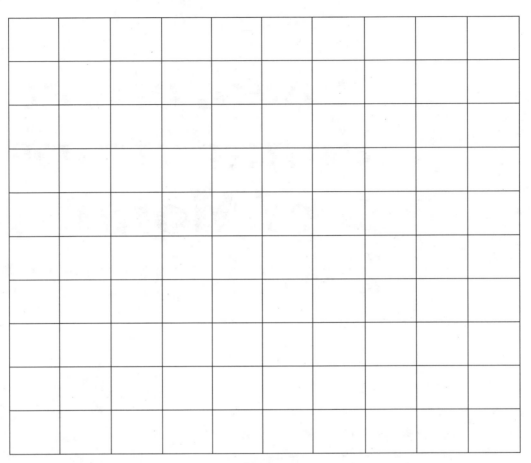

Age in years

From *Learning Activities for Life Span Motor Development Third Edition* by Kathleen Haywood and Nancy Getchell, 2001, Champaign, IL: Human Kinetics.

CHAPTER 2

Theoretical Foundations of Motor Development

Three different paradigms, or worldviews, exist in developmental research: organismic, mechanistic, and contextual. From these paradigms arise three different theoretical viewpoints specific to motor development. These are the maturational, information-processing, and ecological perspectives. Maturationists emphasize biological development, specifically maturation of the central nervous system. Those following the information-processing perspective see the environment as the main force driving motor development. Ecological theorists stress the interactions among all body systems, as well as the inseparable nature of the individual, environment, and task.

Why is acknowledging the different paradigms and theories important? Why can't you just focus in on the "facts"? First of all, you need to understand your own personal paradigm—what you assume happens in terms of motor development across the life span, and more important, the processes to which you attribute change in motor behavior. In addition, as students of motor development you must be able to interpret knowledge of development in light of the perspective of those generating that knowledge. You must identify biases in interpreting data that will result from a certain perspective and realize the benefits and limitations of adopting a single perspective. Professionals may need to combine aspects of several viewpoints to understand and explain global motor behavior. Furthermore, the treatment or teaching methods you choose will be influenced by the assumptions of the various theoretical perspectives. It's certainly good to know why you teach the way you teach! All these reasons make the study of different paradigms and perspectives important.

ACTIVITY 2.1

Determining Paradigmatic Positions on Developmental Questions

Purpose: To be able to distinguish the basic features that define a worldview or paradigm.

Each worldview takes a different position on the "facts"—the changes we observe over time in individuals' motor development. If a researcher adopts a particular worldview, he or she will interpret those facts in a manner consistent with that paradigm. In other words, the paradigm will explain how the facts came about! Sometimes it is difficult to uncover the underlying paradigmatic assumptions of individuals; it is helpful in that regard to practice interpreting facts using the assumptions of each of the different paradigms.

Instructions and Questions

Carefully read the following scenarios. Each one represents motor development "facts" in a different situation.

After carefully reading each scenario, you should analyze each using the different worldviews. Record your answers on record sheet 2.1. Taking the perspective of each worldview, do the following:

1. Describe the underlying assumptions that would help you interpret each specific scenario. Some assumptions may not be relevant in both cases.

2. List the most important pieces of information ("facts") within the scenario.

3. List the additional facts not mentioned or information you as a researcher would collect that would support your point of view.

4. Draw a graph of the data you have or would collect that would support your point of view. Carefully label your x and y axes.

5. Take a position on whether the scenario presents typical or atypical development. Write a summary statement identifying the underlying processes that have resulted in the facts included in the scenarios. Clearly present the differences as described by the different worldviews.

Scenario I

Susan was born on January 1, 2000, with no apparent physical disabilities. By March 2000, she could raise her head while lying in the prone position; and by April, she could lift up on her elbow and turn her head. In August 2000, the infant could sit without support and could support herself on her hands and knees, but did not attempt to crawl. By October, she could pull herself up on the furniture; and by January 2001 she could walk without assistance. At no time during the year did Susan crawl.

Scenario II

As a teenager, Joe played baseball in a recreational league. As an outfielder, he could throw a ball with both force and accuracy. Joe got a job after high school and did not throw a baseball again for 50 years. At age 67, Joe took part in the Senior Olympics. On his first throw, he could throw about half as far as he had as a teenager.

Scenario I

Assumptions

Organismic	Mechanistic	Contextual

Important information				Supplementary information		
Organismic	Mechanistic	Contextual		Organismic	Mechanistic	Contextual
1.	1.	1.		1.	1.	1.
2.	2.	2.		2.	2.	2.
3.	3.	3.		3.	3.	3.

Graph

Organismic	Mechanistic	Contextual

From *Learning Activities for Life Span Motor Development Third Edition* by Kathleen Haywood and Nancy Getchell, 2001, Champaign, IL: Human Kinetics.

(continued)

Summaries

A. Organismic _____

_____

_____

B. Mechanistic _____

_____

_____

_____

_____

C. Contextual _____

_____

_____

_____

_____

Scenario II

Assumptions

Organismic	Mechanistic	Contextual

Important information				Supplementary information		
Organismic	**Mechanistic**	**Contextual**		**Organismic**	**Mechanistic**	**Contextual**
1.	1.	1.		1.	1.	1.
2.	2.	2.		2.	2.	2.
3.	3.	3.		3.	3.	3.

From *Learning Activities for Life Span Motor Development Third Edition* by Kathleen Haywood and Nancy Getchell, 2001, Champaign, IL: Human Kinetics.

(continued)

Graph

| Organismic | Mechanistic | Contextual |

Summaries

A. Organismic _____

_____

_____

B. Mechanistic _____

_____

_____

_____

C. Contextual _____

_____

_____

_____

From *Learning Activities for Life Span Motor Development Third Edition* by Kathleen Haywood and Nancy Getchell, 2001, Champaign, IL: Human Kinetics.

ACTIVITY 2.2

Analyzing Motor Development Information on the World Wide Web

Purpose: To critically examine information sources from the Internet on the topic of motor development.

The World Wide Web can be an incredible resource for any practitioner. Many organizations and advertisers provide information that anyone with a computer can access. It is important to keep in mind that there are few regulations on the World Wide Web; anyone can make almost any claim (whether it is based on research, opinion, or something else). You, as an informed consumer, must examine Web sites carefully and determine the usefulness and accuracy of their information, just as you would with library research. In this learning activity, you will explore the Web and try to determine the theoretical assumptions and underpinnings of various Web sites.

Instructions and Questions

1. Using any Internet browser you choose, enter the term "motor development" on the search engine (e.g., Yahoo, Alta Vista, Lycos). Of the first 10 hits, what are the types of Web sites that you encounter?

2. From your list, pick a Web site that is an advertisement for a motor development product. What is the product and to whom is the product marketed?

3. What are the underlying assumptions of the advertiser regarding motor development? For example, does the advertiser take a maturationist, information-processing, or ecological systems point of view? What leads you to believe this?

4. Pick three other Web sites and repeat this process. Try to pick Web sites that address different issues in motor development (i.e., aging, disabilities, infancy, childhood). Summarize your findings. Are there any trends that you can see regarding motor development and the Internet?

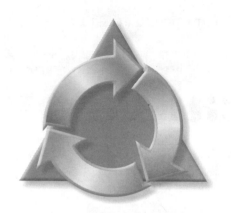

PART II

Physical Growth and Aging

CHAPTER 3

Physical Growth, Maturation, and Aging

The model of constraints is a useful one for the study of motor development because the role of individual, structural constraints in movement during the periods of growth and aging is obvious. The model of constraints demonstrates that changes in any constraint can give rise to a different movement pattern. Movement patterns naturally change during the periods of the life span in that there are great changes in body size, shape, and proportion. For example, think about a 2-year-old boy. How is he able to first jump up off the ground? One month he cannot get both feet to leave the ground together, but the next month he can! Consider that one explanation could be physical growth. The legs are relatively short at birth. They must grow in early life to "catch up" to the head and trunk. So, the legs get bigger as well as stronger, since muscle growth is ongoing. We see, then, that one explanation for advancement in motor skills is physical growth. We can better understand changes in motor development by appreciating the changes in the body that take place with growth and aging. The study of growth and aging is an important subtopic for the study of motor development. In this chapter, we will explore measures of growth and aging; measuring growth and rate of growth; and changes in the body with aging.

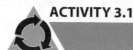

ACTIVITY 3.1

Graphing a Velocity Curve

Purpose: To distinguish between the extent of growth and the rate of growth and to take note of several landmarks in growth highlighted by velocity curves.

When most of us think of charting growth, we think of a *distance curve*. That is, we think of plotting a child's height or weight, perhaps at each birthday in childhood and adolescence. From such a graph we could see *how far* a child had grown at any point in his youth. For example, from a height distance curve we can determine how tall an individual was at any given age (for the plot of an individual person) or what the average height for a group was at any age (if group averages are plotted). The plot tells us other things, too. If the line is going up with age, we know that growth is taking place. If the line is flat, there is no growth. If the slope of the line is steep, the rate of change is rapid; and of course if the line has a gradual slope, the change is moderate. That is, the slope of a distance growth curve can indicate changes in the rate of growth.

If we want to picture the rate of growth in a more dramatic way, we can take the change in growth from a distance curve and plot what is called a *velocity curve*. A velocity curve is a chart plotting the speed or rate of growth against age. A velocity curve can be plotted for any distance measure. Now, you might say, why bother? One reason is that a velocity curve quickly and easily points to certain landmarks in the course of growth. An example of one of these landmarks is a peak in a velocity curve. Velocity curves look very different from distance curves. Whereas a distance curve for growth will rise with age, a velocity curve will have peaks and valleys. A velocity curve peak helps us identify the age at which growth was the fastest. We often call this the age of peak height velocity or peak weight velocity, depending on the growth measure being observed. It is interesting to compare the age at various peak velocities between genders or across other groups.

To get a better feel for what distance and velocity curves represent, plot a velocity curve for height and a curve for weight in this activity.

Instructions

1. Table 3.1 gives the height (in centimeters) attained by a boy on each of his birthdays from 6 to 22 years. Plot these data, making sure height is on the vertical axis and age is on the horizontal axis. You can graph these data by hand on graph paper or with a computer software program, such as Microsoft® Excel®. Submit your graph with record sheet 3.1.

TABLE 3.1

Age	6	7	8	9	10	11	12	13	14	15	16	17	18	19	20	21	22
Ht (cm)	120	125	130	136	143	149	155	164	170	175	178	181	182	183	184	184	184

2. From these height data you should complete the table in record sheet 3.1 on p. 25 showing the change in height from one birthday to the next. That is, determine the increase in height from age 6 to age 7 and enter that for the 6 to 7 interval, and so on. For example, the increase from age 6 to age 7 is 5 cm.

3. When you have completed this table for the change in height, or rate of growth in height, plot these data. An obvious question is where to plot the change for each interval. That is, should you plot the change from 6 to 7 years at 6, at 7, or somewhere in between? The common practice is to plot the change at the midpoint of the time interval. In this case, you would plot the change from 6 to 7 (5 cm) at 6.5 years, the change from 7 to 8 years at 7.5 years of age, and so on. Submit your graph with record sheet 3.1.

4. Table 3.2 shows the growth in weight (in kilograms) for a girl from 5 years to 18 years. Repeat the same steps as with height to create distance and velocity curves for weight. Calculate the change in weight for every age interval, and record your calculations on record sheet 3.1. Plot these data points by hand on graph paper or with a computer software program. Submit your graphs with record sheet 3.1.

TABLE 3.2

Age	5	6	7	8	9	10	11	12	13	14	15	16	17	18
Wt (kg)	16	18	20	23	26	29	33	37	41	46	48	50	51	52

Questions

1. Consider the distance curves. Developmentalists often use the term "age at takeoff" to refer to the age at which an individual enters a period of rapid growth after a period of more steady growth—that is, the age at which one's growth "takes off." What would be the age at takeoff for your two distance curves? Why did you choose these ages as the age at takeoff?

2. Could you determine age at takeoff from your velocity curves? If so, how? If not, why not?

3. Developmentalists also refer to "peak velocities." Examine your velocity curves. Can you determine an age of peak height velocity and an age of peak weight velocity? How did you decide on these ages? Look at the distance curves at the age of peak height velocity and the age of peak weight velocity. Do you know what the place on the distance curve that corresponds to peak velocity is called?

4. Are there any plateaus in your velocity curves? If so, what is the distance curve like in the age spans corresponding to these plateaus?

5. Are there any downslopes in your velocity curves? If so, what is taking place in growth during this time? Hint: Examine the distance curve corresponding to this portion before you answer.

Graphing a Velocity Curve

Change in height

Interval	6-7	7-8	8-9	9-10	10-11	11-12	12-13	13-14	14-15	15-16	16-17	17-18	18-19	19-20	20-21
Change	5														

Change in weight

Interval	5-6	6-7	7-8	8-9	9-10	10-11	11-12	12-13	13-14	14-15	15-16	16-17	17-18
Change													

From *Learning Activities for Life Span Motor Development Third Edition* by Kathleen Haywood and Nancy Getchell, 2001, Champaign, IL: Human Kinetics.

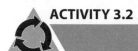

ACTIVITY 3.2

Growth Measures

Purpose: To experience taking physical growth measures and using growth data to obtain even more information about growth status.

There are a number of reasons for tracking the physical growth of children and youths. First and foremost, abnormal growth signals a medical problem that can be subsequently diagnosed and treated such that normal growth can be restored. Abnormal growth can be detected through regular and systematic growth measures. Second, the social relationships of children and youths often revolve around their growth status. For example, the biggest children sometimes assume leadership roles. Too, they might be the "stars" on youth sport teams. Smaller children might be treated by some adults as if they were younger than their actual chronological age, and so on. It is helpful if children and youths know about the course of growth and how their growth is proceeding. Measuring children, along with talking to them about growth patterns, is a useful process. Additionally, growth measurements can teach us a great deal about the normal course of physical growth and the individual variability we can expect within a group.

For growth screenings to be meaningful, measurements must be done accurately, and the measurement techniques must be the same as those used to establish group norms or averages. Standard techniques are described in a number of publications. If you were to be involved in a formal screening program, you would want to obtain a description of the standard technique and follow it carefully. Researching standard techniques is beyond the scope of our activity here, but carefully following the instructions in this chapter will help familiarize you with an accepted measurement technique. It is good to appreciate the discipline and preparation needed to take accurate measurements.

The measures used to assess growth and size are known as *anthropometric* measures. They include height, weight, segment lengths, body breadths at various locations, and circumferences at various locations. Sometimes we use the direct measures in a ratio to illustrate a particular aspect of size. This learning activity gives you some exposure to all of these measures and methods.

Equipment List

Stadiometer, long anthropometer, or wall-mounted tape measure

Skinfold calipers

Breadth or bow calipers

Tape measure

Scale

Instructions and Questions

1. Locate a toddler or child. Record the child's birth date. Then, convert the child's age to a decimal by adding his/her age in years to the number of months since the last birthday divided by 12 months. For example, a child 6 months past his/her 5th birthday is 5.5 years old.

2. You can work with a partner, one of you taking a measurement and the other recording it. Be sure to reverse roles for some measurements. Ideally, you should practice on each other before measuring a child. To be consistent, any measurements you take on only one side of the body should be taken on the right side.

Record all your measurements on record sheet 3.2 on p. 30. *Note:* The assumption here is that you are measuring on metric scales. You can measure on English scales, but be sure that you are consistent since later you will enter your data into some formulas. It is absolutely necessary that all your data be in one scale or the other!

3. You should take three measurements and then average the three to obtain the measurement you will use in later calculations. This minimizes errors in measurement. If one of your three measurements is greatly different from the other two, you might assume that you read the scale incorrectly or wrote the figures incorrectly. In this case, throw out the odd number and average the other two.

4. Measure the individual's *standing height* with the stadiometer (see figure 3.1). Have the individual stand erect against the stadiometer with arms at sides. Ask the individual to take a full breath and then lower the horizontal rule until it touches the crown of the head and is at a right angle with the vertical rule. Record your measurements.

5. Now place a flat stool in front of the measurement scale of the stadiometer and measure the height of the stool. Have the child sit on the stool and measure this *sitting height*, using the same method as with standing height. Later, subtract the stool height from the sitting height you recorded.

6. Weigh the child on the scale with his or her shoes off. Young children might not be good at standing still! Be sure that the child is standing in the middle of the scale's platform when you take the measure.

7. Measure and record the child's head circumference above the eyebrows, using the tape measure (see figure 3.2). Be sure that the child's head is level and that your tape measure is in a horizontal plane.

8. Record the circumference of the child's upper arm, halfway between the shoulder (acromion process) and elbow (olecranon). Make sure the tape measure is perpendicular to the long axis of the arm.

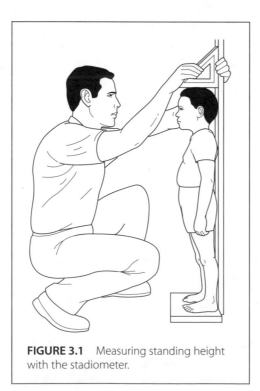

FIGURE 3.1 Measuring standing height with the stadiometer.

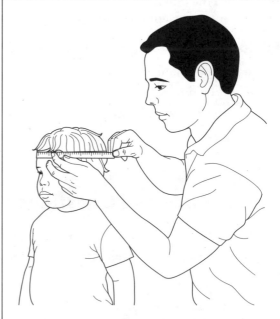

FIGURE 3.2 Measuring head circumference with a tape measure.

9. Measure the shoulder breadth with an anthropometer or bow caliper. Place the arms of the instrument on the lateral (outside) edge of the acromion process. You should palpate the top of the shoulder to find this bony landmark while standing behind the child (see figure 3.3).

10. Measure the hip breadth with the same instrument. Palpate for the top of the iliac crest from behind the child, and place the instrument's arm on the outside edge of the crest.

11. Using skinfold calipers, measure the triceps skinfold. With the arm relaxed at the side, raise a vertical fold of skin on the back of the upper arm, midway between the shoulder (acromion process) and elbow (olecranon), as with the upper arm circumference (see figure 3.4). Place the caliper arms midway between the crest and base of the fold about 1/2 in. (1.3 cm) below the pinch site. Read and record the thickness.

12. Measure the calf skinfold. Mark the inside of the calf (medial surface) at the level of maximum calf circumference. Have the individual place the foot on an elevated surface with the knee flexed at a right angle. Raise a vertical fold of skin just above the mark; then use the skinfold calipers to measure the skinfold thickness, again about 1/2 in. (1.3 cm) below the pinch site, midway between the crest and base of the fold (see figure 3.5). Read and record this number.

13. Now that you have obtained the needed measures, calculate the following ratios. First, divide the shoulder breadth measure by the hip breadth measure and multiply by 100. This ratio represents the trunk build. The larger the number, the more the individual's build is that of broad shoulders and narrow hips. Again, enter your results on record sheet 3.2 on p. 30.

14. Next, calculate the portion of the standing height that is legs (vs. trunk and head). Subtract the individual's sitting height (did you remember to remove the height of the stool?) from his or her standing height. This provides a functional measure of

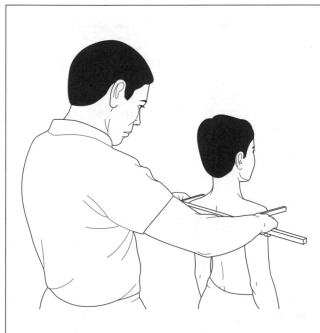

FIGURE 3.3 Measuring shoulder breadth with an anthropometer after first identifying the acromion process.

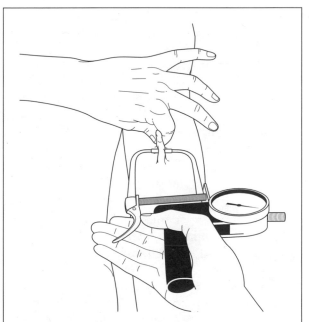

FIGURE 3.4 Measuring the triceps skinfold (a skinfold midway between the shoulder and the elbow) using calipers.

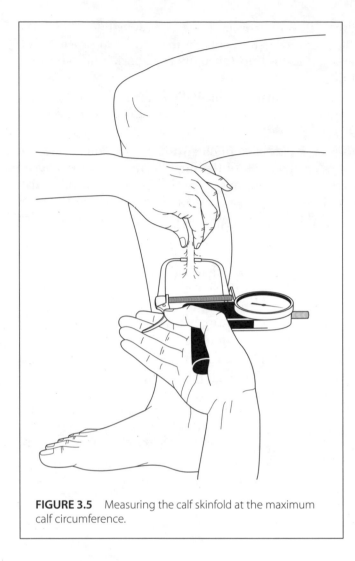

FIGURE 3.5 Measuring the calf skinfold at the maximum calf circumference.

leg length. Divide leg length by standing height and multiply by 100. This provides the percentage of standing height that is the legs. If you obtained 50%, the legs would be exactly one-half of the individual's standing height.

15. It is possible to estimate the portion of the upper arm that is lean tissue versus fat tissue. Use your upper arm circumference and triceps skinfold measures. These measurements must be in the same units. You probably measured skinfold in millimeters and will need to convert to centimeters to match the circumference measure. Multiply your skinfold measure by the value of pi (3.14), and then subtract this value from your upper arm circumference measure. This provides an estimate of the lean circumference of the arm. You can divide lean circumference by overall circumference to obtain the portion of the upper arm that is lean tissue.

16. The calf and triceps skinfolds were selected for this learning activity because researchers have worked out a means to estimate total body fat percentage in children from these two measurements. This means is not a good estimate for adults. Add your calf and triceps measurements in millimeters. Locate this number across the top of one of the two bars in appendix A, depending on whether the individual is a boy or girl. Move straight down to the bottom of the bar to read the percent body fat estimate. The zones these figures fall into are also labeled "very low," "low," and so on. Record both the numerical estimate of percent body fat and the category.

17. Now calculate this individual's body mass index (BMI). Convert the individual's height to *meters* and then square the height. Take the body weight in kilograms and divide body weight by the squared height, or use the chart in appendix B to read the BMI based on the individual's height and weight. Refer also to table B.1 in appendix B to find out which category (underweight, normal weight, etc.) an individual with this BMI would be in. For example, if the BMI is between 21 and 24, the individual is classified as normal weight, although this measure is probably more accurate for adults than children and youths.

18. Consult appendix C for graphs showing how to calculate the stature and weight by age percentiles for boys and girls. Approximate the height and weight percentiles

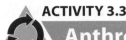

ACTIVITY 3.3
Anthropometric Measurement of an Older Adult

Purpose: To take anthropometric measures on an older adult and use the data to calculate other descriptive measurements.

Growth ends for humans in the late teens or early 20s. But, as most adults can testify, this does not mean that the body maintains its size over the adult years. A variety of extrinsic factors can influence body size, especially weight.

Height is stable through adulthood, aside from very slight increases in trunk length. Stature might decrease in older adulthood because of compression and flattening of the cartilage pads between the spinal vertebrae. Osteoporosis also can result in such a loss of bone density that vertebrae actually collapse and the loss of stature becomes pronounced.

Adults typically start gaining fat weight in their early 20s, almost always as a result of lifestyle changes. Those who exercise regularly and eat wisely, though, often maintain their weight or even gain muscle mass while losing fat weight. Older adults sometimes lose weight, having become so inactive as to lose muscle mass, although loss of appetite accompanying changes in lifestyle can be a factor.

So, extrinsic factors play a larger and larger role as individuals proceed through the adult years and the effects accumulate. As a result there is great variability among adults with regard to how and how much their body size and shape have changed. In this activity, you will take several anthropometric measurements that can be used to calculate other descriptors of body size and composition. These descriptors can be used to compare and contrast individuals across the life span or to observe changes in individuals over their own life span.

Equipment List

Scale

Stadiometer, long anthropometer, or wall-mounted tape measure

Skinfold calipers

Tape measure

Instructions

1. You can work with a partner so that one of you can take a measurement and the other record it. Locate a middle-aged adult and an older adult. You should follow the instructions in activity 3.2 for taking the anthropometric measures needed in this exercise. Record your measurements and calculations on record sheet 3.3 on p. 33.

2. Record each individual's gender and age.

3. Measure each individual's standing height and sitting height.

4. Weigh each person.

5. Record the circumference of the upper arm, and take a triceps skinfold.

6. If time permits, interview both individuals. Ask how they think their bodies have changed since young adulthood. Ask what they think has contributed to those changes, and ask about weekly exercise activities.

7. Using standing and sitting height, calculate the portion of standing height that is legs versus trunk and head. Again, record the results of your calculations on record sheet 3.3 on p. 33.

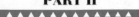
8. Using the upper arm circumference and triceps skinfold, calculate the portion of the upper arm that is lean tissue versus fat tissue. Don't forget to put all your measurements in the same units.

9. Using the height in meters and the weight in kilograms, calculate BMI.

Questions

1. If you completed activity 3.2, use the data from the child you measured in answering these questions. Compare your "subjects" on percentage of height that is leg length. Do you think similarities and differences reflect age or genetic influence on body proportions?

2. Compare your subjects on the portion of the upper arm that is lean tissue. Do you think similarities and differences reflect age, gender, or lifestyle (including exercise activities and diet)?

3. Finally, compare your subjects on BMI. Recall that a BMI between 21 and 24 is considered to be in the "normal" range. Do you think similarities and differences reflect age or lifestyle (again, including exercise activities and diet)?

4. In what ways do you think the body size and composition information you obtained is linked to what the individual said about things that have contributed to changes in the body, especially exercise activities?

RECORD SHEET 3.3

Anthropometric Measurement of an Older Adult

Individual	1					2			
	Gender		Age			Gender		Age	
Measurement #	1	2	3	Average		1	2	3	Average
Standing height	5'1"	5'1"	5'1"						
Sitting height	4'6"	4'6"	4'6"						
Arm circumference	11	11	11						
Triceps skinfold	16	17	18						
Weight	110.2	110.2	110.1						

head circumference 22 in.
shoulder breadth 12.5 in

Calculations

Calculation	Your value
Leg % of height	
Lean tissue % of arm	
Body mass index (BMI)	

From *Learning Activities for Life Span Motor Development Third Edition* by Kathleen Haywood and Nancy Getchell, 2001, Champaign, IL: Human Kinetics.

hip breadth 11.5 in
calf skinfolds 29 mm

CHAPTER 4

Development and Aging of Body Systems

The ecological perspective recognizes that the individual consists of many systems that interact with one another. This interaction is of particular interest during periods of the life span when one or more systems are changing rapidly. Consider that even if only one system changes, its interaction with each of the other stable systems changes and thus changes the individual in many ways! In this chapter we emphasize some of the body systems most involved in physical growth: the skeletal system, the muscle system, and the adipose tissue system. Recall from the introduction to chapter 3 the discussion of a 2-year-old boy learning to jump off the ground. We acknowledged that growth of the legs is a possible explanation for the rather sudden onset of this skill. At the system level, leg growth consists of skeletal and muscle growth. Another explanation, though, could be advancement of the nervous system. Perhaps the nervous system needed to develop to a stage at which movements at the hip, knee, and ankle joints could be coordinated to project the body off the ground. We can see that both whole body growth and system growth can inform our study of motor skill acquisition. In our activities here, we typically will look at change within a single system; but keep in mind that any one system always interacts with the others. Ultimately, we want to be able to consider the changes in many systems, and their interactions, in our study of motor development.

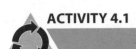

ACTIVITY 4.1

Estimating Skeletal Age

Purpose: To estimate skeletal age by comparing simulated hand and wrist X rays with the simulated standard for an individual of known chronological age.

Physiological maturation is more difficult to assess than physical growth. We cannot see as easily the qualitative advancement in biochemical composition of the body's cells, organs, and systems. Inferences about physiological maturation made on the basis of age alone, size alone, or even age and size together often invite error. A few indicators of physiological maturation are easy to observe, good examples being dental eruption and secondary sex characteristics, but are limited to a narrow portion of the life span.

Skeletal maturation is a reflection of physiological maturation that can be used at any time in the growth period. The most commonly assessed site of skeletal maturation is the hand and wrist. Although an assessment requires a hand and wrist X ray, the result is an exact "maturation" age that can be contrasted with chronological age. The hand and wrist are used because of the large number of bones and sites that can be compared between an individual and a "standard." *A Radiographic Standard of Reference for the Growing Hand and Wrist* by S.I. Pyle, a book of standards that is available, contains many X rays for various chronological ages throughout the growth period. Comparisons can be made on the roundish carpal bones of the wrist, the epiphyseal growth plates of the long bones of the hand and fingers, and the epiphyseal growth plates of the forearm bones.

Although you are not likely to have skeletal maturation information about the individuals with whom you work, being familiar with the process highlights some important lessons about individual differences. Children of a given age can vary widely in physiological maturation. The activities of this exercise demonstrate how we know this to be the case.

Instructions

1. Study the simulated X ray of the hand and wrist of a 6-year-old girl in figure 4.1. This simulated X ray is the standard for a girl 6.0 years old. Note the number of wrist bones (carpals) ossified, the extent of their ossification, and the extent of ossification at the epiphyseal growth plates located at the ends of the long bones of the hand (metacarpals and phalanges) and forearm (radius and ulna). The extent of ossification at an epiphyseal growth plate typically is seen by how completely the end of the bone is ossified. Initially there is a small area of ossification that is not even as wide as the bone shaft. With continued skeletal maturation the epiphysis is seen as larger and as having more of the eventual, adult shape.

2. Now study the simulated X ray in figure 4.2 and compare it to the standard in figure 4.1 for the same features. Record the results of your comparison on record sheet 4.1 on p. 37. Enter *m* for "more" if the number of ossification centers or the extent of ossification is more than the standard, *l* for "less," or *s* for "same."

3. Do the same for the simulated X ray in figure 4.3; then answer the following questions.

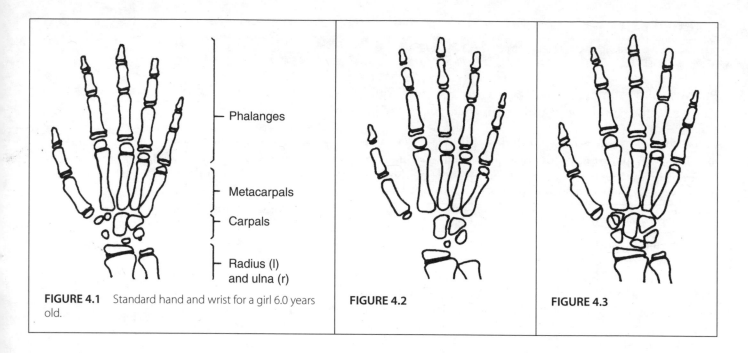

FIGURE 4.1   Standard hand and wrist for a girl 6.0 years old.

FIGURE 4.2

FIGURE 4.3

Questions

1. From your assessment as recorded in record sheet 4.1, is the child whose X ray appears in 4.2 more or less physiologically mature than the standard for a 6-year-old? That is, is the skeletal age for the child of figure 4.2 younger or older than 6.0 years? On what do you base your answer? Can you reach a conclusion about the chronological age of this child? Why or why not?

2. From your assessment as recorded in record sheet 4.1, is the child whose X ray appears in figure 4.3 more or less physiologically mature than the standard for a 6-year-old? What can you say about this child's chronological age in relation to skeletal age, if anything?

3. The standard X ray in figure 4.1 depicts the skeletal development of a girl at 6.0 years of age. Would the standard X ray of a boy at 6.0 years chronological age be likely to show more or less skeletal development? Why?

4. It is possible for a normally developing but early- or late-maturing child to be as much as 1 to 1.5 chronological years ahead or behind the skeletal maturation shown in a standard. Assume you are working with a group of boys between 10.0 and 11.0 years of age, chronologically. What could the range of skeletal ages be among this group of boys?

For example, they might indicate that they stopped playing tennis because they could no longer find tennis partners or because they moved to new locations; or they might indicate that they changed diet on the advice of a physician.

Questions

1. How does each interviewee compare to the typical patterns described in the introduction to this activity?

2. If one or both of your interviewees differs from the typical profile, identify any factors that seem to be responsible for their individual patterns.

Skeletal, Muscle, and Adipose System Changes Over the Life Span

Interview With 45- to 60-Year-Old

Age _____ Sex _____

1. Body weight at various points of the life span:

   Young adulthood   Present

2. Any osteoporosis? Had bone scan?

3. Any changes in height? Any fractures?

4. Any changes in muscle mass? Any muscle-building activities?

5. Any changes in fat weight? In distribution of fat weight? Any activities influencing fat weight?

6. What were the diet and exercise patterns? Any changes in these patterns?

Interview With 60- to 80-Year-Old

Age _____ Sex _____

1. Body weight at various points of the life span:

   Young adulthood   Present

2. Any osteoporosis? Had bone scan?

3. Any changes in height? Any fractures?

4. Any changes in muscle mass? Any muscle-building activities?

5. Any changes in fat weight? In distribution of fat weight? Any activities influencing fat weight?

6. What were the diet and exercise patterns? Any changes in these patterns?

From *Learning Activities for Life Span Motor Development Third Edition* by Kathleen Haywood and Nancy Getchell, 2001, Champaign, IL: Human Kinetics.

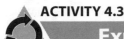

ACTIVITY 4.3

Exploring Skeletal Injuries in Youth Sport

Purpose: To research the risks to the growing skeleton associated with the participation of children and youths in sport programs, and to decide on policies for youth sport programs.

The skeleton begins as a cartilage model and ossifies over the growth period. In the long bones of the body the shaft ossifies first, during the prenatal period. Further growth in length is achieved at the ends of the shaft, called the epiphyseal plate, growth plate, or pressure epiphysis. This epiphyseal plate is a cartilage zone with layers of cells in varying stages of preparation for the addition of bone to the end of the bone shaft. Bone is laid down at the epiphyseal plates until the cartilage zone disappears and growth of that bone stops.

Some bones grow until late adolescence. The various epiphyseal plates throughout the body close at different ages. These ages are younger in early maturers and of course older in late maturers. Since girls as a group mature earlier than boys, bone growth typically stops at younger ages in girls than in boys.

An injury that disturbs the blood supply to the cartilage zone where new cells are being formed and nourished could disturb the growth process at the epiphyseal plate. If the injury is to a left leg, for example, while the right leg is undisturbed, the result could be differences in bone length between the right and left limbs. In this case, treatment typically would involve surgery to repair the blood supply to the injured limb. The younger an individual is at the time of injury, the greater the potential for significant repercussions. Though broken bones typically heal well and quickly in children receiving proper treatment, epiphyseal plate injuries are of great concern.

There also are growth sites on the bones where muscle tendons attach to the bone. These are called traction epiphyses. The traction epiphyses are subject to acute injuries as well as to overuse injuries from repetitive, forceful pulling by the muscle tendon.

Fortunately, the number of epiphyseal injuries resulting from sport participation, in contrast to automobile or home accidents, is small. Yet parents, teachers, coaches, therapists, and program organizers should pay particular attention to reducing the risk of such injuries in youth sport programs. They should put into place program guidelines that protect young participants yet allow participants to enjoy the sport.

Instructions

1. Form a group of approximately five classmates.
2. Research sport injuries in childhood and adolescence using the World Wide Web or by searching an electronic database available through a college or university library; find at least three types of sport injuries and record the following information about each on record sheet 4.3 on p. 43.
3. Identify whether the risk is from an acute incident or from repetitive overuse.
4. Identify whether the risk is associated with a particular sport.
5. Determine whether or not children and youths are more susceptible to this injury than adults (that is, whether the injury is related to immaturity of the growing skeleton).
6. In the cases of repetitive overuse, note whether a particular level (amount per unit of time) of training is associated with increased risk.

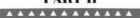

7. Note any evidence you find of steps taken by program organizers to reduce risk (this could be in the form of protective equipment or equipment modifications in the case of acute injuries, or training/participation limitations in the case of over-use injuries).

8. Next, your group should play the role of a committee established to create training and competition guidelines for a competitive youth swimming program sponsored by a community center. Two individuals should play the role of parents, one should play the role of the program director, one the role of a pediatrician, and one the role of a college coach. You should adopt the perspective you anticipate each of these would bring to the discussion.

9. Write a set of guidelines for the swimmers participating in this program. The guidelines should cover the length of the competitive and training seasons, the length of practices, the number of practices in a week without a scheduled competition, and the number of practices in a week with a scheduled competition. Submit your guidelines along with record sheet 4.3.

Questions

1. What guideline or guidelines were the most difficult for your group to write? Why? What different points of view or considerations did you debate before you arrived at the final version? What guideline was the easiest to agree on? Why?

Sport Injuries in Youths

#1, Injury: _____

Acute incident or repetitive overuse?

Sport or sports where observed:

Are youths more susceptible than adults? Why?

Level of training that increases risk:

Evidence of attempts to reduce risk:

#2, Injury: _____

Acute incident or repetitive overuse?

Sport or sports where observed:

Are youths more susceptible than adults? Why?

Level of training that increases risk:

Evidence of attempts to reduce risk:

#3, Injury: _____

Acute incident or repetitive overuse?

Sport or sports where observed:

Are youths more susceptible than adults? Why?

Level of training that increases risk:

Evidence of attempts to reduce risk:

From *Learning Activities for Life Span Motor Development Third Edition* by Kathleen Haywood and Nancy Getchell, 2001, Champaign, IL: Human Kinetics.

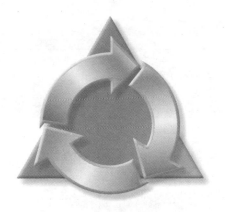

PART III
▲▲▲▲▲▲▲▲▲▲▲

Motor Development

CHAPTER 5

Early Motor Development

The first year of life for an infant represents a period of rapid change in motor development. Infants are thrust into a strange, new world, one with a plethora of new sensations and experiences. In the short span of about 1 year, infants' movements change from seemingly spontaneous, weak, reflexive, and reactive to goal directed and independent. As observers of motor development, we must ask, What changes do infants go through? Further, we want to determine how interacting constraints allow certain behaviors to emerge in typically developing children. For example, an infant must have sufficient muscular strength (individual, structural constraint) to pull herself up to a standing position; at the same time, she must be motivated to stand (individual, functional constraint), have a firm surface to hold her body weight (environmental constraint), and have something to pull up on (task constraint). Most typically, infants will attain common motor milestones in a universal order, although there are individual differences in the timing of attainment. Therefore, people working with infants should know what behaviors usually occur in infants, as well as the developmental order of attainment of these behaviors.

ACTIVITY 5.1

Identifying Constraints During Infancy and Toddlerhood

Purpose: To identify the changing constraints that exist during infancy and toddlerhood, and to relate them to specific motor achievements.

Infancy is a time of rapid change. Many different systems, such as the muscular and nervous systems, mature at their own rates but at the same time interact with all other systems. As observable movements, these changes are often termed "motor milestones."

The attainment of a milestone indicates a unique interaction of various constraints that allows the particular behavior to emerge. For each infant, the rate at which motor milestones appear (and to a certain extent, the type of milestone—related to locomotion, reaching, or posture, for example) for one infant can differ from that for other infants. This indicates that particular constraints may act as rate limiters, or controllers, for a given infant. When a critical value of that rate limiter is at last reached, the infant will achieve the motor milestone or skill.

Instructions: Part A

The photos on pages 47 and 48 are of one infant as she progresses through infancy and toddlerhood. The pictures are not in a particular order.

1. Put the photos in order of attainment—that is, which skill was most likely attained first, second, and so on (see table 5.2 in your textbook)? Record your answers on record sheet 5.1a on p. 49. You can use both milestone scales (the Bayley scales and the Shirley scales); however, keep in mind the relative order rather than the ages associated with attainment.

2. For each photo, list which constraints are most likely to encourage this skill.

3. For each photo, list which constraints are most likely acting as rate limiters to the attainment of future skills.

4. Discuss the role of constraints in the attainment of motor skills. Explain why the milestones were attained in a particular order, and how constraints change throughout infancy and toddlerhood.

Following is an example using the two sample photographs below. The order of attainment and constraints are bolded. The picture on the left (example A) shows the infant sitting on her own. The picture on the right (example B) shows the infant supported by a pillow, thrusting her arms and legs.

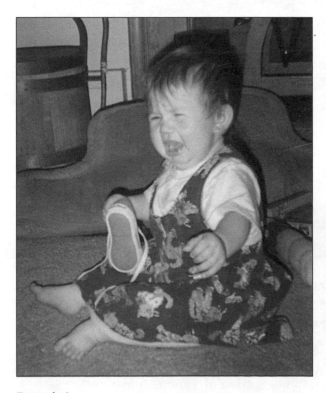

Example A

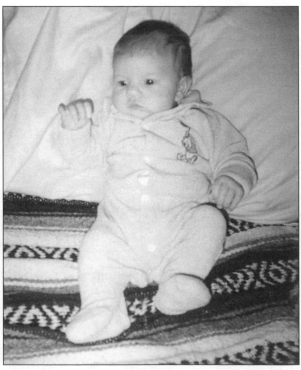

Example B

1. The order of attainment is **B then A.**
2. In example B, **arm and leg strength** as well as **neurological maturation** allows for arm and leg thrusting. The **supporting pillow** encourages a more upright posture, which allows the infant to see in front and may motivate her to thrust her arms and legs even more. In example A, **neck and trunk strength** allows the infant to sit upright on her own. **Motivation (or displeasure)** also appears to be playing a role in this infant's emergent behaviors.
3. In example B, **neck, back, and trunk strength** limits the infant's ability to sit. She needs support in order to attain even a slight upright posture. In example A, **leg strength** limits her ability to pull to stand, and **balance and posture** prevent this infant from walking.
4. Use the discussion to reflect on constraints in infancy, such as why certain milestones come before others, how individual constraints change, and the importance of environmental and task constraints.

Now try this with figures 5.1 through 5.6.

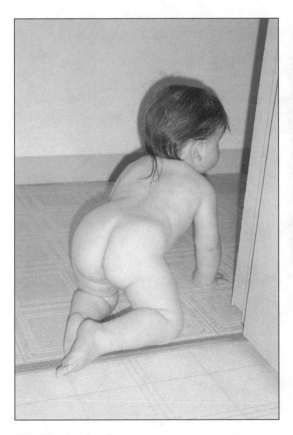

FIGURE 5.1 Crawling.

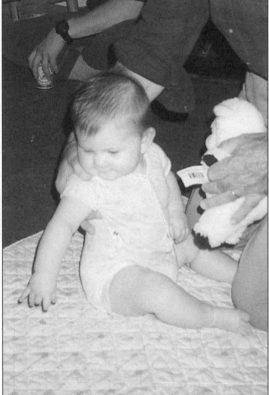

FIGURE 5.2 Sitting with support.

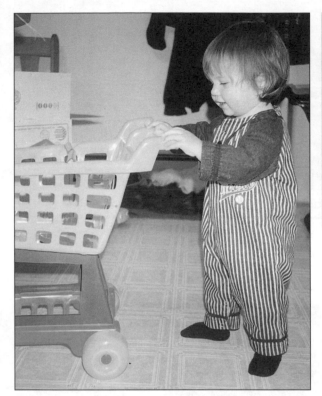

FIGURE 5.3 Walking with support.

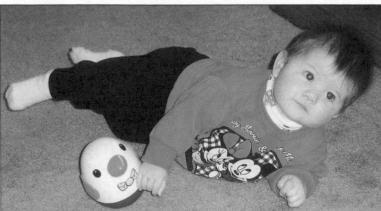

FIGURE 5.4 Rolling.

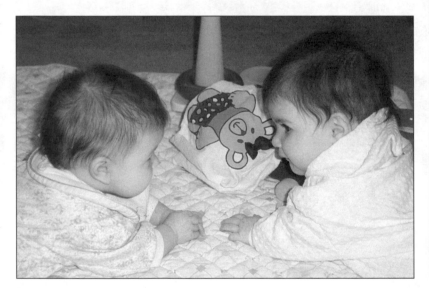

FIGURE 5.5 Lifting head and shoulders.

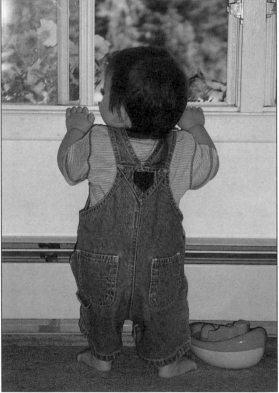

FIGURE 5.6 Pulling to stand.

A. Order of Motor Milestone Attainment

First	Second	Third	Fourth	Fifth	Sixth

B. Constraints That Encourage Milestones in Each Picture

First	Second	Third	Fourth	Fifth	Sixth
1.	1.	1.	1.	1.	1.
2.	2.	2.	2.	2.	2.

C. Constraints That Discourage Milestones in Each Picture (Rate Limiters)

First	Second	Third	Fourth	Fifth	Sixth
1.	1.	1.	1.	1.	1.
2.	2.	2.	2.	2.	2.

D. Discussion

_____

_____

_____

_____

_____

From *Learning Activities for Life Span Motor Development Third Edition* by Kathleen Haywood and Nancy Getchell, 2001, Champaign, IL: Human Kinetics.

Instructions: Part B

The chapter 5 folder on your CD-ROM contains video clips of several infants at different points in infancy and toddlerhood. The clips are not in a particular order. You will approach part B just as you did part A, by watching the clips and then determining developmental order and different constraints.

1. Put the video clips in developmental order—that is, rank the clips from early to late infancy/toddlerhood. Record your answers on record sheet 5.1b.
2. For each video clip, list which constraints are most likely to encourage this skill.
3. For each video clip, list which constraints are most likely acting as rate limiters to the attainment of future skills.
4. Discuss the role of constraints in the attainment of motor skills. Explain why the milestones were attained in a particular order, and how constraints change throughout infancy and toddlerhood.

A. Order of Motor Milestone Attainment

First	Second	Third	Fourth	Fifth	Sixth

B. Constraints That Encourage Milestones in Each Video Clip

First	Second	Third	Fourth	Fifth	Sixth
1.	1.	1.	1.	1.	1.
2.	2.	2.	2.	2.	2.

C. Constraints That Discourage Milestones in Each Video Clip (Rate Limiters)

First	Second	Third	Fourth	Fifth	Sixth
1.	1.	1.	1.	1.	1.
2.	2.	2.	2.	2.	2.

D. Discussion

_____

_____

_____

_____

_____

From *Learning Activities for Life Span Motor Development Third Edition* by Kathleen Haywood and Nancy Getchell, 2001, Champaign, IL: Human Kinetics.

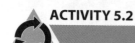

ACTIVITY 5.2

Observing the Motor Milestones

Purpose: To observe the motor milestone skills in an infant under 1 year of age and to assess the rate of motor development in an infant by comparison to norms.

The rudimentary motor skills leading to locomotion are acquired in a relatively consistent sequence, making it possible to identify a common age range for acquisition of each skill. Of course, there is some variation in the rate of appearance of the motor milestones. The rate of physical maturation and a variety of environmental factors play roles in individual variability. Several normative scales exist for comparing the age at which an infant acquires a given skill with the average age and range of ages when typically developing infants acquire the skill. Infants who acquire skills late thus can be identified and monitored by professionals.

In this activity you will observe an infant under 1 year of age and consider his/her motor development in relation to norms (see textbook chapter 5, pp. 98-99, for more on norm-referenced scales). Remember that every great athlete started by acquiring these same rudimentary skills.

Equipment List

A toy ring

A building block

Instructions

1. Your instructor will arrange for you to work with an infant.

2. Obtain the background and general information, particularly age. Record the information on record sheet 5.2 on pages 54 to 55. Enter "NA" (not available) for any information you cannot get. The APGAR score is a newborn assessment given directly after delivery. Scores range from 0 to 5, with the higher numbers indicating a more positive newborn assessment.

3. Use the Motor Milestone Observation Guide on page 55. Starting with the first item, position the infant as directed. On record sheet 5.2, enter *O* for observed if the infant exhibits the behavior. Enter an *R* for reported by caretaker. You need not administer the entire scale. If an infant does not show several behaviors in a row and is obviously developmentally younger than the age range for an item, you may stop. The guide provides an average age range so that you can compare the performance of your infant with age norms for performance of these infant motor behaviors.

Questions

1. How far has the infant progressed along the sequence of motor milestones? Does the baby's chronological age match the average age range for the skills you observed? What can you conclude about the infant's motor development?

2. When the baby was lifted from a back-lying position, what was the response of the head? Could the baby sit independently or with support? What postural responses did the infant make in the sitting position? Could the baby stand with support or alone? What postural responses did the infant make when standing?

3. How did circumstances such as the infant's reaction to you or the time lapse since the last feeding or nap affect performance of the infant's motor skills? Did the baby's clothing seem to restrict the execution of any skills? What types of constraints are these factors?

4. Given that this might have been your first observation of infant motor development and that you observed the infant only briefly, how confident are you that your results are accurate? What would you say in explaining your results to the infant's caretaker?

5. Consider the individual, environmental, and task constraints affecting the infant. How did these interact to allow motor behavior to emerge for this infant? What changes in constraints might allow for different behaviors to emerge?

Background and General Information

Today's date _____ Infant's birth date _____ Infant's age ____.____ months

APGAR score at birth _____ Weight at birth _____

Was infant full-term or premature? Full term _____ Premature _____ No. of weeks _____

Special medical problems _____

_____

Is parent/caretaker present? **Y   N**   Time of day _____

How does infant react to you (cries, smiles, etc.)? _____

Hours since last feeding _____ Next feeding expected at _____

Hours since last nap _____ Next nap expected at _____

Clothing that may restrict the infant's movement _____

_____

Infant's general level of alertness/activity _____

Constraints _____

_____

_____

_____

Notes _____

_____

_____

_____

_____

From *Learning Activities for Life Span Motor Development Third Edition* by Kathleen Haywood and Nancy Getchell, 2001, Champaign, IL: Human Kinetics.

(continued)

Motor Milestone Observation Guide

Observed (O) or reported by caretaker (R)	Starting position	Action	Typical age range (weeks)
_____	On belly	Makes crawling motions	1-12
_____	On back	Kicks legs and thrusts arms	1-8
_____	Held upright	Holds head erect	3-16
_____	On side	Rolls to back	3-20
_____	On belly	Pushes with arms to elevate chest	3-20
_____	On hard surface	Sits with help	4-20
_____	Held upright	Holds head steady	4-20
_____	On hard surface	Sits with slight help	8-24
_____	On back	Rolls to side	8-28
_____	On back	Pulls to sit with help	16-32
_____	On hard surface	Sits alone briefly	16-32
_____	On hard surface	Sits alone 30-40 seconds	20-32
_____	On back	Rolls to front	16-40
_____	On hard surface	Sits alone	20-36
_____	On belly	Scoots around	20-44
_____		Crawls on hands and knees	20-44
_____		Moves on hands and feet	20-44
_____	Sitting	Scoots	20-44
_____	Sitting	Pulls to standing position	20-48
_____	Standing	Stands by furniture	24-48
_____	Standing	Walks with help	28-48
_____	Standing	Sits down	28-56
_____	Standing	Stands alone	36-64
_____	Standing	Walks alone	36-68
_____	Sitting on floor	Stands up	36-72

From *Learning Activities for Life Span Motor Development Third Edition* by Kathleen Haywood and Nancy Getchell, 2001, Champaign, IL: Human Kinetics.

Adapted from N. Bayley, 1969, Motor scale. In *Bayley Scales of Infant Development* (New York: Psychological Corporation).

ACTIVITY 5.3

Observing Toddler Behavior

Purpose: To observe motor development in early childhood and to use a criterion-referenced scale for assessment of motor development.

A normative scale such as that used in activity 5.2 is useful in showing how a baby performs in comparison to a reference group of infants. An alternative purpose in assessing skill acquisition during early childhood is to determine whether a child can do a certain skill. When this is the goal, it is appropriate to use a criterion-referenced assessment scale. The child's performance is compared to a predetermined level of mastery rather than with the scores of other children. This assessment permits parents and educators to design an instructional program aimed at fostering the further mastery of basic skills.

Two sections of the Geismar-Ryan Infant-Toddler Developmental Checklist are used here to give you experience with a criterion-referenced scale (see textbook chapter 5, pp. 98-99, for more information on criterion-referenced scales). One section assesses gross-motor and the other section fine-motor activities. You will identify those skills a child performs with competence, those skills in which no competency is demonstrated, and those skills in which competency is just emerging. Skills in the latter two categories would be the basis for planning learning activities for the child, were this your purpose.

Equipment List

Small toy	Small rocking chair	Push/pull toy
Ball	Small bottle	String and beads
Building blocks	Cardboard book	Bowl and jars with lids
Small chair	Pushcart	Balance beam
Cheerios cereal	Crayon and paper	Pegboard and pegs
Puzzle or formboard	Safety scissors	

Instructions

1. Your instructor will make arrangements for you to visit a preschool program or nursery school. You should administer this scale to a toddler over 1 year of age but younger than 5. Ask your instructor whether the equipment needed is available at the school or whether you must bring some items.

2. Obtain as much general and background information on the child as possible, and enter it on record sheet 5.3 on pages 58 through 60.

3. Review the scale beforehand. Become familiar with the tasks so that you can instruct the child, set up equipment, or provide opportunity for the child to demonstrate the behavior.

4. Items at the beginning of each scale are easier and therefore more appropriate for younger children, whereas later items are more difficult and more suitable for older children. You may skip items obviously easy for the child. For example, items 1 to 4 on the gross-motor section might be skipped if you are working with a 4-year-old.

CHAPTER 6

Principles of Motion and Stability

Skilled performers often share many of the same movement characteristics across a variety of activities. This is no coincidence! These performers have learned, one way or another, to use the physical laws of nature to their benefit. In this section, we will explore these principles of motion and stability in addition to the process of attaining motion and stability.

When children and novices perform motor skills, their initial attempts at skills seem to be inefficient and jerky. They may move the body in separate, discrete steps rather than as a whole movement. They often try to optimize one aspect of the movement (such as balance) at the expense of another (such as speed) in order to increase the likelihood of success. As individuals become more proficient at skills, their movements become smoother and more efficient—often, their movement patterns change entirely! Many of the improvements individuals achieve during childhood are due to increases in body size and strength and therefore their ability to produce force. Yet size and strength alone do not account for how children progress from un-skilled to skilled performance. Part of the process of change comes from mastering and exploiting the principles of motion and stability. In fact, all individuals can use these principles to their advantage, in athletic performances and activities of daily living.

ACTIVITY 6.1

Searching for Movement Similarities and Differences in Various Skills

Purpose: To determine movement similarities and differences in proficient performances of various sport skills, which will indicate specific mechanical principles that are used to optimize performance.

When proficient athletes perform skills, they try to optimize their unique individual constraints with specific equipment and task requirements, all within a particular environment. It would seem that each sport has a set of unique movement patterns that represents the best way to take advantage of mechanical principles. To a certain extent, this is true; at the same time, though, movement patterns in various activities involve many common elements that are part of a proficient performance. The major mechanical principles involved in efficient, skilled locomotion include the application and absorption of force, action and reaction, and stability and balance. Knowledge of these principles will allow us to generalize across locomotor skills. The following learning activity will help you to determine the purpose of movements in proficient performance in relation to the principles of motion and stability, and to find both general and specific elements of these skills.

Instructions

On pages 64 through 67 are pictures of eight different athletes participating in sports (examples A-H). For each photo, answer the following questions. Use the photo of the martial artist and the sample answers on the following page to guide you through questions 1 and 2. The principles of motion and stability are bolded.

Questions

1. Determine the goal of the particular movement, both in general (i.e., "score a goal") and specifically (i.e., "kick the ball with both force and accuracy into the net").

2. Based on each picture and your description of the goal of the movement, determine which of the principles of motion and stability the athletes use in their performance.

3. What movements do athletes perform in common to take advantage of the principles? Place the pictures in groups based on their similarities, and describe the general movements that are common to the athletes in each group.

4. What movements specific to a skill do athletes perform that take advantage of the principles of motion and stability? For each picture, describe a unique movement by the athlete that aids in proficient performance of that particular skill.

5. Reflect on the common elements among the athletes. How could you teach, coach, or train individuals in some general way so that they can learn and understand how to optimize movements based on these principles?

1. The general goal of a sparring match in the martial arts is to hit your opponent more times than he hits you. Specifically, a martial artist needs to generate force quickly, as well as to deliver blows accurately in order to score points.

2. The martial artist must move his limbs quickly through a full range of motion to generate as much **torque** (rotational force) as possible. He optimizes this **by fully extending his limb.** By applying the maximized force in a short time, he can apply **impulse** to his opponent.

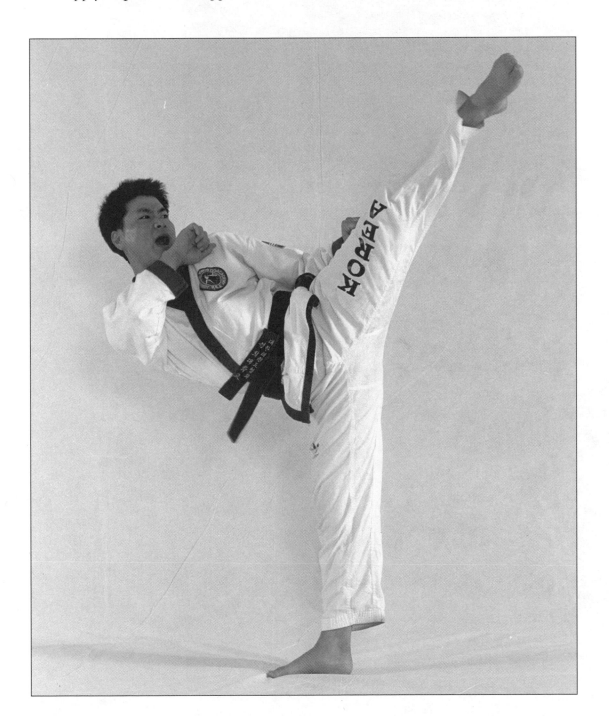

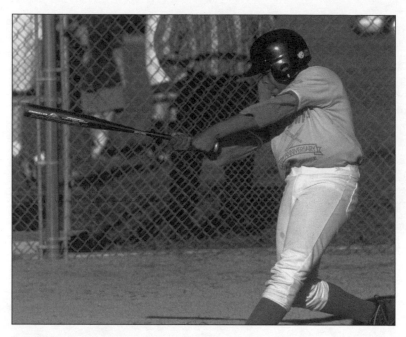

EXAMPLE A

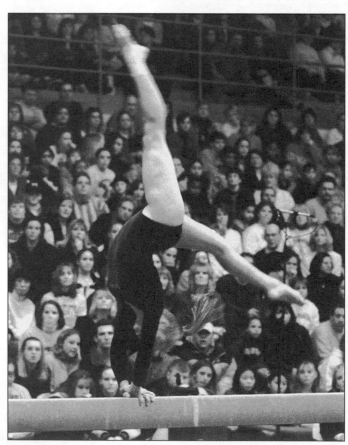

EXAMPLE B

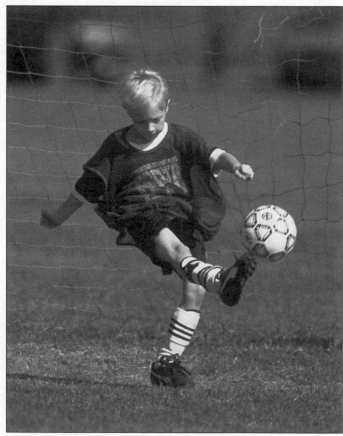

EXAMPLE C

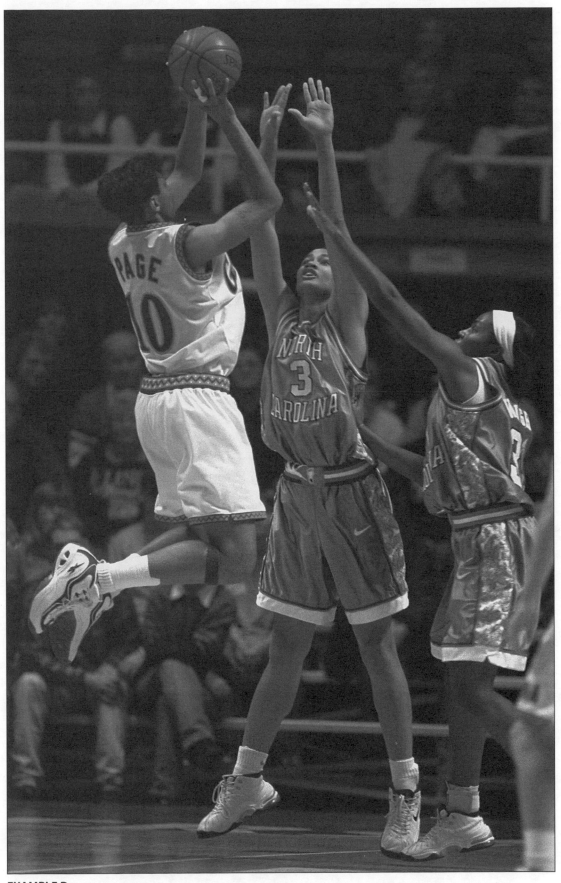

EXAMPLE D

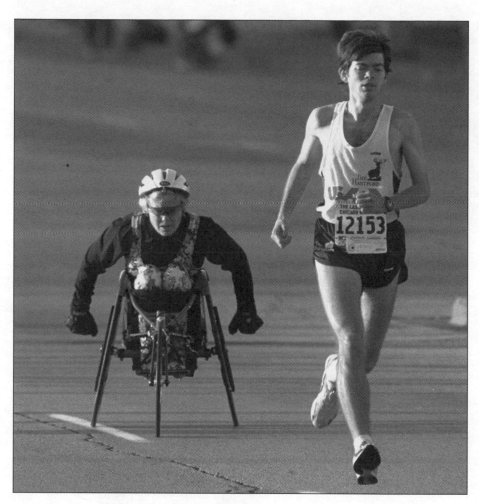

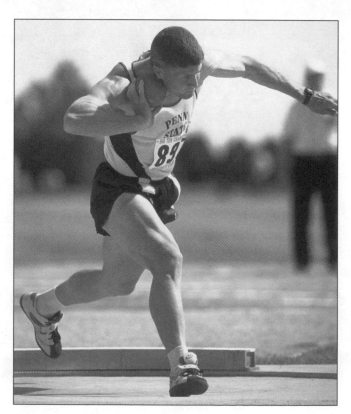

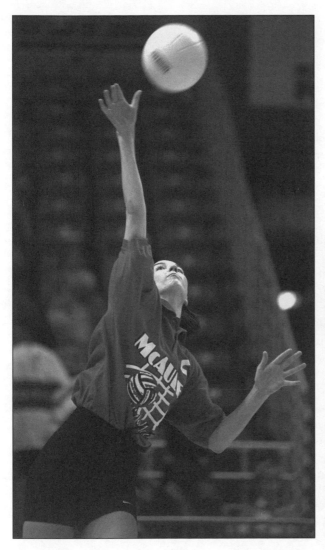

EXAMPLE G

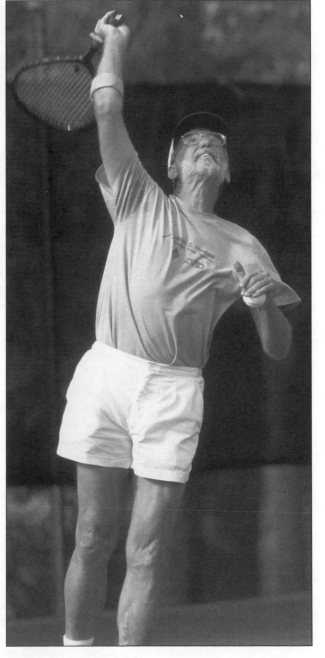

EXAMPLE H

Developmentally Sequencing Locomotor Movements Based on the Principles of Motion and Stability

Purpose: To examine developmental changes in movements based on the principles of motion and stability, to improve the ability to evaluate movements, and to rank and sequence locomotor performances on the basis of these developmental changes.

When observing locomotion, teachers, coaches, or therapists are often called on to describe and analyze movements then determine the developmental status of individuals on the basis of this analysis. These professionals can use either process or product measures to determine success on a task; however, only qualitative analysis provides a valid indication of developmental status. To a novice at movement analysis, this may seem like a somewhat daunting task—each skill may have many different key elements, and to watch and describe each may seem impossible. However, the task becomes much simpler if there exists some sort of general developmental continuum on which the observer can place the movement. Fortunately, the principles of motion and stability provide such a continuum, which acts as a road map across the development of locomotion as well as other skills.

As you may recall from chapter 6 in the textbook, there are certain mechanical principles that shape how individuals interact with the environment when performing a task. For example, gravity pulls us toward the earth at all times; because of this, we follow a parabolic path when we leave the ground (e.g., in hopping, running, jumping). The qualitative changes in motor performance that occur during childhood reflect changes in the interaction between the growing child and the environment. As they progress, children, beginners, or relearners select movement patterns that more and more often optimize the movement product, consistent with the principles of motion and stability.

Instructions

1. You will observe four different movement sequences for the locomotor skills of hopping and standing long jump. These movement sequences are on your CD-ROM. Select the folder labeled Chapter 6 and then the folder labeled Hopping. When you are finished with hopping, move on to the folder labeled Standing Long Jump. There are two sets of four clips for each of the locomotor skills. You will work with Group A and your partner will work with Group B.

2. View each clip in your set carefully. Watch each individual's performance; in particular, look for developmental differences in movement form. Identify the most important principles of motion and stability that affect the performance of each task and record them on record sheets 6.1 and 6.2 on pp. 70 and 71.

3. Rank the clips from least to most developmentally advanced, using the principles of motion and stability as a guide. Record your sequences on record sheets 6.1 and 6.2.

4. Provide a rationale for your sequence, justifying your choices based on the ability of the mover to take advantage of the principles you identified. For example, a new walker uses a **wide base of support** to optimize balance. An older child or adult uses a much smaller base of support, which provides more mobility.

5. Work with your partner, who has observed the other set of video clips for each skill. Together, you have ranked two different sets of videos from least to most developmentally advanced. Now, you will work together with all eight clips. Analyze all the sequences, and for each skill combine the two sets so that you rank all eight clips from least to most developmentally advanced. Record these sequences on record sheets 6.1 and 6.2.

6. Using your new developmental rankings, revise your rationales.

7. Compare your rankings and rationales with those of other pairs of students. Use this information to create a developmental continuum for each task based on the optimization of principles of motion and stability. In other words, describe the changes from early to proficient performance.

Questions

1. Did your partner and classmates choose similar or different mechanical principles in each of the skills? On what did they base their selection of principles?

2. What developmental similarities could you identify across the different locomotor tasks?

Hopping

Important Priniciples of Motion and Stability

Your Development Ranking of Movement Sequences

Least advanced			Most advanced

Your Partner's Ranking of Movement Sequences

Least advanced			Most advanced

Combined Rankings

Least advanced						Most advanced	
1	2	3	4	5	6	7	8

Developmental Continuum

From *Learning Activities for Life Span Motor Development Third Edition* by Kathleen Haywood and Nancy Getchell, 2001, Champaign, IL: Human Kinetics.

Standing Long Jump

Important Principles of Motion and Stability

Your Developmental Ranking of Movement Sequences

Least advanced			Most advanced

Your Partner's Ranking of Movement Sequences

Least advanced			Most advanced

Combined Rankings

Least advanced						Most advanced	
1	2	3	4	5	6	7	8

Developmental Continuum

From *Learning Activities for Life Span Motor Development Third Edition* by Kathleen Haywood and Nancy Getchell, 2001, Champaign, IL: Human Kinetics.

ACTIVITY 6.3

Developmentally Sequencing Ballistic Skills Based on the Principles of Motion and Stability

Purpose: To examine developmental changes in ballistic skills based on the principles of motion and stability, to improve the ability to evaluate movements, and to rank and sequence ballistic performances on the basis of these developmental changes.

Ballistic skills offer a different challenge to observers of movement. Unlike locomotor skills, which tend to be performed continuously, ballistic skills occur in one quick motion. This requires that observers become well acquainted with the developmental progression of the particular skill they are to analyze. This becomes a much simpler task after one has determined the salient principles of motion and stability related to the skill and has ranked performances of the skill based on their use. The basic procedure you will follow is the same one you used in the previous learning activity. However, the most important principles of motion and stability are different between the two types of skills.

Instructions

1. You will observe four different movement sequences for two ballistic skills: overarm throw for force and kicking. On your CD-ROM, select the folder labeled Chapter 6. Start by clicking on Overarm Throw. After you complete your work with Overarm Throw, click on the folder labeled Kicking. There are two sets of four clips for each locomotor skill. You will work with Group A and your partner will work with Group B.

2. View each clip in your set carefully. Watch each individual's performance; in particular, look for developmental differences in movement form. Identify the most important principles of motion and stability that affect the performance of each task and record them on record sheets 6.3 and 6.4 on pp. 74 and 75.

3. Rank the clips from least to most developmentally advanced, using the principles of motion and stability as a guide. Record your sequences on record sheets 6.3 and 6.4.

4. Provide a rationale for your sequence, justifying your choices based on the ability of the mover to take advantage of the principles you identified.

5. Work with your partner, who has observed the other set of video clips for each skill. Together, you have ranked two different sets of videos from least to most developmentally advanced. Now, you will work together with all eight clips. Analyze all the sequences, and for each skill combine the two sets so that you rank all eight clips from least to most developmentally advanced. Record these sequences on record sheets 6.3 and 6.4.

6. Using your new developmental rankings, revise your rationales.

7. Compare your rankings and rationales with those of other pairs of students; create a developmental continuum for each task based on the optimization of principles of motion and stability. In other words, describe the changes from early to proficient performance.

Questions

1. The skills in this section are described as "ballistic," or free-falling. What important environmental constraint affects how far the object will be projected? How do the movers in the clips developmentally change to account for this environmental constraint?

2. What sort of developmental changes do you see in the regulation of posture and balance?

Overarm Throw for Force

Important Principles of Motion and Stability

Your Developmental Ranking of Movement Sequences

Least advanced			Most advanced

Your Partner's Ranking of Movement Sequences

Least advanced			Most advanced

Combined Rankings

Least advanced						Most advanced	
1	2	3	4	5	6	7	8

Developmental Continuum

From *Learning Activities for Life Span Motor Development Third Edition* by Kathleen Haywood and Nancy Getchell, 2001, Champaign, IL: Human Kinetics.

Kicking

Important Principles of Motion and Stability

Your Developmental Ranking of Movement Sequences

Least advanced			Most advanced

Your Partner's Ranking of Movement Sequences

Least advanced			Most advanced

Combined Rankings

Least advanced			Most advanced				
1	2	3	4	5	6	7	8

Developmental Continuum

From *Learning Activities for Life Span Motor Development Third Edition* by Kathleen Haywood and Nancy Getchell, 2001, Champaign, IL: Human Kinetics.

ACTIVITY 6.4

Developmentally Sequencing Manipulative Skills Based on the Principles of Motion and Stability

Purpose: To examine developmental changes in manipulative skills based on the principles of motion and stability, to improve ability to evaluate movements, and to rank and sequence manipulative performances on the basis of these developmental changes.

Just like ballistic skills, manipulative skills tend to be discrete and performed quickly. This leads to difficulty in observation and analysis without some sort of developmental continuum based on specific principles of motion and stability. Again, you will develop such a continuum while honing your skills of observation. The basic procedure you will follow is the same one you used in the previous two learning activities. However, the most important principles of motion and stability are different from those for the previous two types of skills.

Instructions

1. You will observe four different movement sequences for the locomotor skill of catching. On your CD-ROM, select the folder labeled Chapter 6 and then the folder labeled Catching. There are two sets of four clips for catching. You will work with Group A and your partner will work with Group B.

2. View each clip in your set carefully. Watch each individual's performance; in particular, look for developmental differences in movement form. Identify the most important principles of motion and stability that affect the performance of the task and record them on record sheet 6.5 on p. 78.

3. Rank the clips from least to most developmentally advanced, using the principles of motion and stability as a guide. Record your sequence on record sheet 6.5.

4. Provide a rationale for your sequence, justifying your choices based on the ability of the mover to take advantage of the principles you identified.

5. Work with your partner, who has observed the other set of video clips for the skill. Together, you have ranked two different sets of videos from least to most developmentally advanced. Now, you will work together with all eight clips. Analyze both sequences, and combine the two sets so that you rank all eight clips from least to most developmentally advanced. Record this sequence on record sheet 6.5.

6. Using your new developmental rankings, revise your rationale.

7. Compare your rankings and rationale with those of other pairs of students. Use this information to create a developmental continuum for catching based on the optimization of principles of motion and stability. In other words, describe the changes from early to proficient performance.

Questions

1. Look at the developmental continuums that you created in activities 6.2 through 6.4. Are there any similarities that you can find among them? What can you say in general about the development of proficiency in sport skills?

2. Take the role of a teacher, coach, therapist, or trainer. How could you use the information you've obtained in activities 6.1 through 6.4 to help you improve the motor performance of the individuals with whom you work? Try to come up with three or four practical applications based on your analyses.

Catching

Important Principles of Motion and Stability

Your Developmental Ranking of Movement Sequences

Least advanced			Most advanced

Your Partner's Ranking of Movement Sequences

Least advanced			Most advanced

Combined Rankings

Least advanced						Most advanced	
1	2	3	4	5	6	7	8

Developmental Continuum

From *Learning Activities for Life Span Motor Development Third Edition* by Kathleen Haywood and Nancy Getchell, 2001, Champaign, IL: Human Kinetics.

CHAPTER 7

Development of Human Locomotion

Humans use many forms of locomotion over the life span. Newborns have no locomotion whatsoever, but within the first year of life they have rolled, scooted, crawled, and crept through their environment! At about 1 year of age children walk, and in the next few years they add running, galloping, jumping, and hopping. Somewhat later they add skipping. In later childhood, adolescence, and adulthood, individuals often combine locomotor skills for a specific activity. These activities include sport and dance, but also can include work-related activities, such as building construction or military service. Later in life, individuals may have to change their locomotor patterns, to run or walk more slowly or even with the aid of a walker or cane. Some forms of locomotion may no longer be possible.

At any point of the life span, the locomotor skills of an individual reflect the interaction of constraints. To be sure, many locomotor skills emerge when growth or the development of specific systems advances to a point to permit that movement; that is, systems, acting as individual, structural constraints, might be *rate-controlling* systems in the development of a locomotor skill. In the older portion of the life span, changes in systems might also function as rate-controlling systems to bring about decline in locomotor performance. Of course, the environment can always constrain locomotor skills. Ice can cause us to walk more carefully, hot sand can cause us to run more quickly, or a narrow pathway can cause us to sidestep. Task goals can influence locomotion. Reaching the other end of a balance beam without falling off constrains us to walk differently than strolling to class.

Often, parents, teachers, coaches, and therapists want to assess an individual on locomotor skills. They might want an assessment of what the individual can do in an environment conducive to proficient performance and with a goal of optimal performance. At other times, they might prefer an assessment of locomotor skill in a specific environment or with a certain goal. In this chapter, you will use assessment tools to observe runners, jumpers, and hoppers. These tools

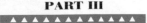
are based on the developmental sequences. That is, the qualitative changes that children make in acquiring locomotor skills can be used as categorizations for individuals of all ages. When an individual does not perform at the highest developmental level, it may be that the individual never achieved the highest developmental level; or it may be that an aspect of the individual, the environment, or the task constrains the individual's movement. The assessment allows us to label a movement pattern to universally represent it to others familiar with the assessment tool.

In this chapter you will assess developmental sequences from several different sources. You will start with photographs so that you can begin to identify specific qualitative features of the locomotor skills. You will progress to a guided assessment, which is provided on the CD-ROM. Finally, after developing the skills you need to accurately assess developmental levels, you will assess locomotor skills from the CD-ROM on your own.

ACTIVITY 7.1
Assessing the Developmental Levels of Runners

Purpose: To gain experience in assessing the developmental levels of runners.

Running shares many movement features with walking. Both have a 50% phasing relationship of the legs; that is, each leg moves through the same cycle, but is a half cycle different in timing than the other leg. The arms move in opposition to the legs in both running and walking: as one leg moves forward, the arm on the opposite side of the body moves forward. A twisting action of the trunk facilitates the step of both locomotor skills. What is different, of course, is that in running an individual has a period of flight, when neither foot is in contact with the ground. Toddlers typically begin to run about 6 or 7 months after they begin to walk. Adults who maintain their running skills and who remain free from diseases and injuries that affect locomotion can run well into older adulthood.

Developmental changes in running, from the time toddlers start to run to the time adolescents become proficient in running, were identified long ago. These developmental trends have been proposed as a series of step-by-step changes, but no one has validated these steps as developmental stages. Here we will use a hypothesized developmental sequence as an assessment tool. The sequence for the leg action in running has three steps. Runners who have only a minimal period of flight and run rather straight-legged, such that the knee of the leg swinging forward (the recovery leg) does not even bend to a right angle, are in the lowest step (minimal flight). Runners who have a longer stride, with a recovery leg that tucks to a knee angle of at least 90°, but who have lateral movement of the legs (cross from side to side), are in the second step (crossover swing). Runners who have a long, full stride when running fast and who drive the legs efficiently forward, with the legs staying in the sagittal (forward-backward) plane, are in the highest step (direct projection).

The sequence for arm action in running has four steps. Runners who hold their arms up, in what is called a middle or high "guard" position, are in the lowest step (high or middle guard). Runners who swing their arms, but swing them together rather than in opposition, are in the second step (bilateral arm swing). Runners who swing the arms in opposition to the legs, but who swing in an oblique plane, laterally and across the body, are in Step 3 (oblique arm swing). Runners who swing the arms in opposition and drive them essentially backward and forward (in the sagittal plane) are in the highest step (opposition, sagittal plane).

Most movement skills occur quickly, and fast movements can be difficult to observe accurately if we have not practiced doing so. A tool that helps novice observers is an observation plan. That is, if observers plan ahead what critical positions and movements to watch for, they can more quickly categorize the performer they are observing. An observation plan for running is provided in this activity, based on the three levels of leg action and four levels of arm action just described. By presenting a series of questions, first for the legs and then for the arms, the plan directs you to watch certain movements and positions. By answering the questions, you eventually arrive at the runner's developmental level or category for each component. A checklist is provided so that once you arrive at that level, you can check the appropriate step number. This is basically the method we will use to observe all the locomotor skills, starting here with running.

Instructions

1. In this activity you will categorize runners by their development levels of running. When categorizing runners viewed in photos or on video, assume that the runner has been instructed to run as fast as possible. Use the Hypothesized Developmental Sequence for Running (table 7.1) and the observation plan on pages 83 and 84 to guide your decisions on the runner's leg and arm action. Begin by categorizing the runner shown in the sequential still photos of figure 7.1 on page 83. Use the observation checklist (record sheet 7.1 on p. 85) to record your answers. Record the designation of the photos (name or photo or video number) on the checklist. Record the runner's age and the date of observation. Also, record the type of observation—photographs. Follow the observation plan to decide the level of the runner for first the leg action and then the arm action. Place a check mark on the corresponding line on the checklist. When finished, translate your check marks into a step number in the summary profile at the bottom of the list.

2. You will repeat the process just described using two different sets of video clips from the CD-ROM. Select the folder labeled Chapter 7 and then the folder labeled Running. Work through the two examples in Set A. You can use slow motion as much as necessary. The program will prompt you to watch for the critical elements, just as in the observation plan. After completing Set A, categorize the examples in Set B. Label a column on record sheet 7.1 for each video example. You will have to follow the observation plan yourself this time. Follow the observation plan to decide the level of each runner, first for the leg action and then for the arm action. Place a check mark on the corresponding line on record sheet 7.1. When finished, translate your check marks into a step number in the summary profile at the bottom of the column. You might not be able to make the final judgements about whether arm and leg motions are in the forward-backward plane, since the video clips present only a side view.

3. After categorizing the photos and videos, arrange to categorize one or several children directly. When doing direct observations, you are responsible for giving runners instructions. Direct them to run as fast as possible but at a speed that is safe for the environment in which they are moving. Allow them to warm up prior to your assessment. You should observe them from two positions: side view (at a right angle from their running path) and front or rear view (directly in front of or behind them).

4. Follow the observation plan to decide the level of each runner, first for the leg action and then for the arm action. Place a check mark on the corresponding line on the checklist. When finished, translate your check marks into a step number in the summary profile at the bottom of the column. You might see runners use the

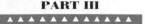
movement pattern characteristic of more than one level as you observe. If so, use the movement corresponding to the point of the run at which the runner has achieved his or her top speed (rather than when the runner starts up or slows down), and use the movement pattern you see most often.

Questions

1. Did runners tend to be at the same step number for the legs and the arms, or did they tend to be at different steps? Cite one or two examples from your checklist.

2. Among the runners you observed, was there an older runner who was at a lower level in one or both body components than a younger runner? Describe any such occurrence.

3. On your direct observation of runners, did you notice any runners who used movements characteristic of more than one level? How often did this occur?

4. Consider the environmental and task constraints for your direct observation. Choose a constraint that, if you had changed it, would likely have changed the movement pattern, and therefore the level, of a runner. Indicate the body component(s) that would change and how it (they) would change.

5. Which method of observation (photos, videos, etc.) did you find the easiest for running? Which did you find the hardest? Why? What are the advantages and disadvantages of each?

TABLE 7.1	
Hypothesized Developmental Sequence for Running	
Leg component	
Step 1	Minimal flight. The running step is short and flat-footed. On the recovery swing forward, the leg is rather stiff.
Step 2	Crossover swing. The stride is long, and the recovery leg knee flexes to at least a right angle. The leg action, though, has lateral movements wherein the legs swing out and in during the recovery.
Step 3	Direct projection. The stride is long, and the recovery leg tucks to swing forward. The legs project directly backward on takeoff and swing directly forward for the touchdown.
Arm action	
Step 1	High or middle guard. The arms are both held up at waist to shoulder level and move very little as the legs stride forward and back.
Step 2	Bilateral arm swing. The arms swing; but they are coupled, moving forward and backward together.
Step 3	Opposition, oblique. The arms drive forward in the opposition pattern, moving forward and backward with the opposite leg, so that one arm is moving forward while the other is moving backward. The arms, though, swing across the chest or out to the side, in a plane oblique to the plane of movement.
Step 4	Opposition, sagittal. The arms swing forward and back in the opposition pattern and stay nearly in the sagittal (or forward-backward) plane of movement.

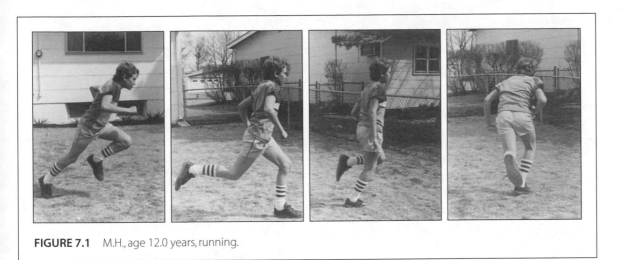

FIGURE 7.1 M.H., age 12.0 years, running.

OBSERVATION PLAN FOR RUNNING

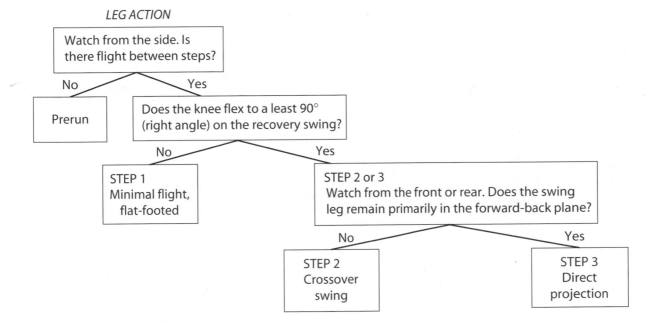

LEG ACTION

Watch from the side. Is there flight between steps?

No → Prerun

Yes → Does the knee flex to a least 90° (right angle) on the recovery swing?

No → STEP 1 Minimal flight, flat-footed

Yes → STEP 2 or 3 Watch from the front or rear. Does the swing leg remain primarily in the forward-back plane?

No → STEP 2 Crossover swing

Yes → STEP 3 Direct projection

(continued)

(continued)

ARM ACTION

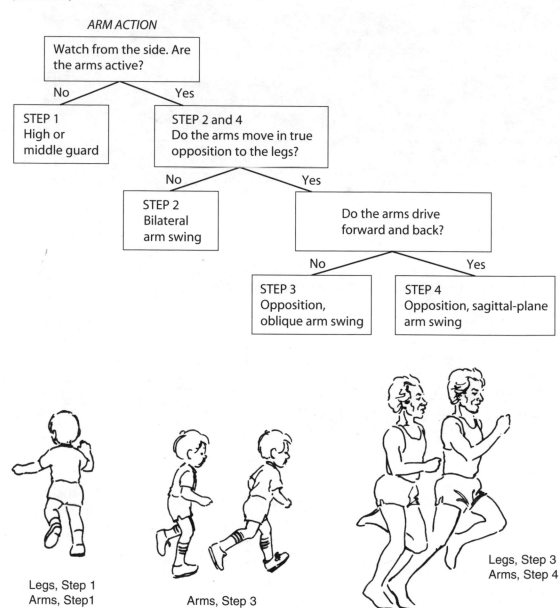

Watch from the side. Are the arms active?

No → STEP 1
High or middle guard

Yes → STEP 2 and 4
Do the arms move in true opposition to the legs?

No → STEP 2
Bilateral arm swing

Yes → Do the arms drive forward and back?

No → STEP 3
Opposition, oblique arm swing

Yes → STEP 4
Opposition, sagittal-plane arm swing

Legs, Step 1
Arms, Step1

Arms, Step 3

Legs, Step 3
Arms, Step 4

sequential still photos of figure 7.2 on page 88. Use the observation checklist (record sheet 7.2 on p. 91) to record your answers. Record the designation of the photos on the checklist under "name." Fill in the jumper's age and the date of observation. Also, record the type of observation—photographs. Follow the observation plan to decide the level of the individual, first for the leg action and then for the arm action. Place a check mark on the corresponding line on the checklist. When finished, translate your check marks into a step number in the summary profile at the bottom of the column.

2. You will repeat the process already described using two different sets of video clips from the CD-ROM. Select the folder labeled Chapter 7 and then the folder labeled Jumping. Work through the two examples in Set A. The program will prompt you to watch for the critical elements of the standing long jump, just as in the observation plan. After completing Set A, categorize the examples in Set B. Label a column on record sheet 7.2 on page 91 for each video example. Just as with activity 7.1, you will have to follow the observation plan yourself this time. Follow the observation plan to decide the level of each jumper, first for the leg action and then for the arm action. Place a check mark on the corresponding line on record sheet 7.2. When finished, translate your check marks into a step number in the summary profile at the bottom of the column.

3. After categorizing the photos and videos, arrange to categorize one or several children directly. When doing direct observations, you are responsible for giving jumpers instructions. Direct them to jump as far as possible. Make sure that the jumping surface is clear of rocks and other debris that may cause injury. Allow the children to warm up prior to your assessment. You should observe the jumpers from the side view (at a right angle from their jumping path). Follow the observation plan to decide the level of each jumper, first for the leg action and then for the arm action. Place a check mark on the corresponding line on the checklist. When finished, translate your check marks into a step number in the summary profile at the bottom of the column. You might see jumpers use the movement pattern characteristic of more than one level in different jumps. If so, use the movement pattern you see the most often (modal level). For example, if you observe a jumper for five jumps, and three of her jumps are at one level and two at another, categorize the jumper at the level observed for three jumps.

Questions

1. Did jumpers tend to be at the same step number for the legs and the arms, or did they tend to be at different steps? Cite one or two examples from your checklist.

2. Among the jumpers you observed, was there an older jumper who was at a lower level than a younger jumper in one or both body components? Describe any such occurrence.

3. On your direct observation of jumpers, did you notice any jumpers who used movements characteristic of more than one level? How often did this occur?

4. Consider the environmental and task constraints for your direct observation. Choose a constraint that, if you had changed it, would likely have modified the movement pattern, and therefore the level, of a jumper. Indicate the body component(s) that would change and how it (they) would change.

5. Which method of observation (photos, videos, etc.) did you find the easiest for jumping? Which did you find the hardest? Why? What are the advantages and disadvantages of each?

TABLE 7.2

Developmental Sequence for the Standing Long Jump Takeoff

Leg action component

Step 1	One-foot takeoff. From the beginning position the jumper steps out with one foot. There usually is little preparatory leg flexion.
Step 2	Knee extension first. The jumper begins to extend the knee joints before the heels come off the ground, resulting in a jump that is too vertical to achieve maximum horizontal distance.
Step 3	Simultaneous extension. The jumper extends the knees at the same time the heels come off the ground.
Step 4	Heels up first. The jump begins with the heels coming off the ground; then the knees extend. The jumper appears to start the takeoff by tipping forward.

Arm action component

Step 1	No action. The arms are stationary. After takeoff they may "wing" (shoulder girdle retracts).
Step 2	Arms swing forward. The arms swing forward at the shoulder from a starting position at the sides. The arms also might swing out to the side (abduct at the shoulder).
Step 3	Arms extend, then partially flex. The arms extend back together during leg flexion, then swing forward together at takeoff. Arm swing never reaches a position overhead.
Step 4	Arms extend, then fully flex. The arms extend back together during leg flexion, then swing forward to a position overhead.

Reprinted, by permission, from K.M. Haywood and N. Getchell, 2001, *Life Span Motor Development,* 3rd ed. (Champaign, IL: Human Kinetics), 131.

Adapted from J.E. Clark and S.J. Phillips, 1985, A developmental sequence of the standing long jump. In *Motor development: Current selected research,* Vol. 1, edited by J.E. Clark and J.H. Humphrey (Princeton, NJ: Princeton Book), 76-77. Copyright © 1985 by Princeton Book Company, Publishers. Reproduced by permission of Princeton Book Company, Publishers.

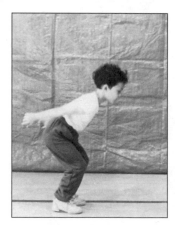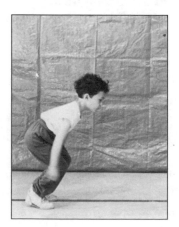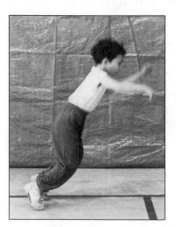

FIGURE 7.2   L.H., age 3.2 years, long jumping.

OBSERVATION PLAN FOR THE STANDING LONG JUMP

LEG ACTION

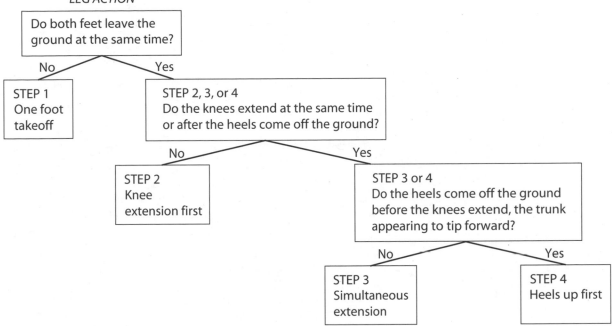

Do both feet leave the ground at the same time?

No → STEP 1 — One foot takeoff

Yes → STEP 2, 3, or 4 — Do the knees extend at the same time or after the heels come off the ground?

No → STEP 2 — Knee extension first

Yes → STEP 3 or 4 — Do the heels come off the ground before the knees extend, the trunk appearing to tip forward?

No → STEP 3 — Simultaneous extension

Yes → STEP 4 — Heels up first

Arms swing forward

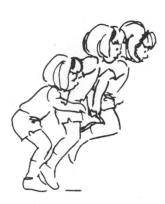

Feet leave ground together

Simultaneous extension

Legs, Step 3
Arms, Step 2

Arms extend then fully flex

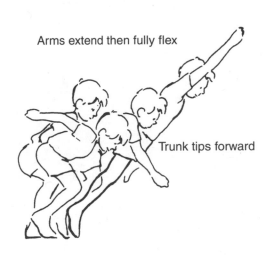

Trunk tips forward

Feet leave ground together

Heels up first

Legs, Step 4
Arms, Step 4

(continued)

(continued)

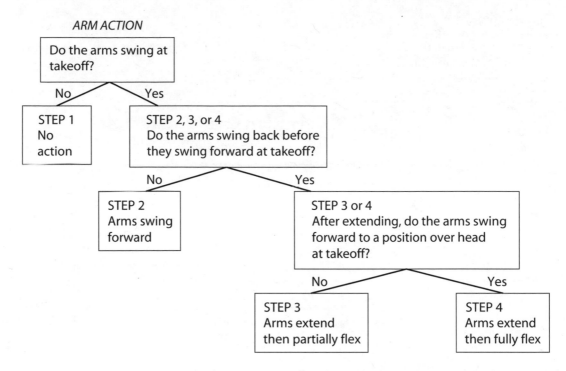

ARM ACTION

Do the arms swing at takeoff?

No — Yes

STEP 1
No
action

STEP 2, 3, or 4
Do the arms swing back before
they swing forward at takeoff?

No — Yes

STEP 2
Arms swing
forward

STEP 3 or 4
After extending, do the arms swing
forward to a position over head
at takeoff?

No — Yes

STEP 3
Arms extend
then partially flex

STEP 4
Arms extend
then fully flex

Assessing the Developmental Level of the Standing Long Jump

Observation Checklist: Jumping

Observation number	1	2	3	4	5	6	7
Jumper's name, photo, or video number							
Jumper's age, if known							
Date							
Observation type*							
Component							
Leg							
Step 1 One-foot takeoff							
Step 2 Knee extension first							
Step 3 Simultaneous extension							
Step 4 Heels up first							
Arm							
Step 1 No action							
Step 2 Arms swing forward							
Step 3 Arms extend then partially flex							
Step 4 Arms extend then fully flex							
Summary profile							
Leg							
Arm							

*Codes for observation type: D = direct; P = photographs; F = film; V = video; S = slow motion.

From *Learning Activities for Life Span Motor Development Third Edition* by Kathleen Haywood and Nancy Getchell, 2001, Champaign, IL.: Human Kinetics.

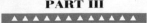

ACTIVITY 7.3

Assessing the Developmental Levels of Hoppers

Purpose: To gain experience in assessing hoppers.

Hopping is the locomotor movement wherein movers project their bodies into the air taking off on one foot and then landing on that same foot. Most often, hoppers execute a series of hops, although they can hop in place or travel through space. Many of the principles of stability and motion that we see applied by proficient hoppers are the same as those applied by proficient runners and jumpers. For example, the arm opposition displayed by proficient runners is displayed by proficient hoppers. Use of the arms to help propel oneself from the ground is seen in both proficient jumpers and hoppers. As you practice assessing hoppers, look for similarities among the locomotor assessments. This will help you identify themes that will improve your accuracy and speed in assessment.

The developmental sequence for hopping has a progression for leg action and a progression for arm action (see table 7.3 on p. 94). At the two lower steps, the "swing" leg, or nonhopping leg, actually does not swing at all. Step 1 leg action is a momentary flight of the body, produced more by a pulling up of the leg than by a forceful exertion on the support surface. Step 2 leg action appears to be a "fall and catch" in which the body leans forward and minimal knee and ankle extension produce the hop. At the two higher steps, the swing leg does swing back and forth and assists in projecting the body off the ground. At Step 3 the range of swing leg motion is somewhat limited, as is knee and ankle flexion, in preparation for the takeoff thrust. At Step 4, the swing leg moves through a large range and leads projection from the ground. The support, or hopping, leg joints flex on landing so that forceful and full extension can project the body off the ground.

Arm action in hopping has five developmental steps. In the lower three, the arms move together. We call this bilateral action. In Step 1 the arms are held bilaterally but are inactive. In Step 2 they react, usually to a loss of balance. They might make winging movements prior to takeoff. In Step 3 the arms assist the hop, pumping up and down as the hopper moves. At the two higher levels, the arms are no longer coupled. In Step 4 the arm opposite the swing leg moves back and forth, as in running, but the other arm is held to the front or side. At the most advanced level, Step 5, both arms move in opposition to the legs, much as in running. The range of movement, though, depends on the speed and distance of the hopping. Be sure to review table 7.3 before conducting your assessments.

As with running and jumping, you should use the observation plan for hopping to guide your observations. Begin with leg action and focus on the movement to which the plan directs you. Move through the plan, making your decisions until you arrive at a step for that particular hopper.

Instructions

1. In this activity you will categorize children for their development levels of hopping. When categorizing hoppers viewed in photos or on video, assume that the individual has been instructed to hop from one place to another. Be aware that very young hoppers might not be able to traverse a distance but will instead hop in place. Use the Developmental Sequence for Hopping (table 7.3) and the observation plan (pp. 95-96) to guide your decisions on the hopper's leg and arm action. Begin by categorizing the individual shown in the sequential still photos of figure 7.3 on p. 95. Use the observation checklist (record sheet 7.3 on p. 97) to record

your answers. Record the designation of the photos on the checklist under "name." Fill in the hopper's age and the date of observation. Also, record the type of observation—photographs. Follow the observation plan to decide the level of the individual, first for the leg action and then for the arm action. Place a check mark on the corresponding line on the checklist. When finished, translate your check marks into a step number in the summary profile at the bottom of the list.

2. You will repeat the process described earlier using two different sets of video clips from the CD-ROM. Select the folder labeled Chapter 7 and then the folder labeled Hopping. Work through the two examples in Set A. The program will prompt you to watch for the critical elements of the hop, just as in the observation plan. After completing Set A, categorize the examples in Set B. Label a column on record sheet 7.3 (p. 97) for each video example. Just as with the previous two activities, you will have to follow the observation plan yourself this time. Follow the observation plan to decide the level of each hopper for first the leg action and then the arm action. Place a check mark on the corresponding line on record sheet 7.3. When finished, translate your check marks into a step number in the summary profile at the bottom of the column.

3. After categorizing the photos and videos, arrange to categorize one or several children directly. When doing direct observations, you are responsible for giving hoppers instructions. Direct them to hop from a start position to some finish position you designate. Make sure the environment is safe and the hopping surface is clear of rocks and other debris that may cause injury. You should observe the hoppers from the side view (at a right angle from their hopping path). Follow the observation plan to decide the level of each hopper, first for the leg action and then for the arm action. Place a check mark on the corresponding line on the checklist. When finished, translate your check marks into a step number in the summary profile at the bottom of the column. You might see hoppers use the movement pattern characteristic of more than one level as you observe. If so, use the movement corresponding to a time when the hopper has achieved his or her top speed (rather than when the hopper starts up or slows down), and use the movement pattern you see the most often (modal level). For example, if a child hops five times from start to finish, and three of the hops are at one level and two at another, categorize the hopper at the level observed for three hops.

4. Assess hoppers first when they hop on the preferred, or chosen, leg. Then, ask at least one of your hoppers to switch legs, hopping on the other leg, and repeat the assessment. Often, hoppers are at a different developmental level on their nonpreferred legs.

Questions

1. Did hoppers tend to be at the same step number for the legs and the arms, or did they tend to be at different steps? Cite one or two examples from your checklist.

2. Among the hoppers you observed, was there an older hopper who was at a lower level than a younger hopper in one or both body components? Describe any such occurrence.

3. On your direct observation of hoppers, did you notice any hoppers who used movements characteristic of more than one level? How often did this occur? Describe which movements you saw.

4. Consider the environmental and task constraints for your direct observation. Choose a constraint that, if you had changed it, would likely have altered the movement

pattern, and therefore the level, of a hopper. Indicate the body component(s) that would change and how it (they) would change.

5. Was your hopper at different developmental levels for the preferred and nonpreferred legs? Was the difference one level or more than one level? Was the difference in leg action, arm action, or both? Describe the differences.

TABLE 7.3

Developmental Sequence for Hopping

Leg action

Step 1	Momentary flight. The support knee and hip quickly flex, pulling (instead of projecting) the foot from the floor. The flight is momentary. Only one or two hops can be achieved. The swing leg is lifted high and held in an inactive position to the side or in front of the body.
Step 2	Fall and catch; swing leg inactive. Body lean forward allows minimal knee and ankle extension to help the body "fall" forward of the support foot and then quickly catch itself again. The swing leg is inactive. Repeat hops are now possible.
Step 3	Projected takeoff; swing leg assists. Perceptible pretakeoff extension occurs in the hip, knee, and ankle in the support leg. There is little or no delay in changing from knee and ankle flexion on landing to extension prior to takeoff. The swing leg now pumps up and down to assist in projection. The range of the swing is insufficient to carry it behind the support leg when viewed from the side.
Step 4	Projection delay; swing leg leads. The weight of the child on landing is now smoothly transferred along the foot to the ball [of the foot] before the knee and ankle extend to takeoff. The support leg nearly reaches full extension on the takeoff. The swing leg now leads the upward-forward movement of the takeoff phase, while the support leg is still rotating over the ball of the foot. The range of the pumping action in the swing leg increases so that the swing leg passes behind the support leg when viewed from the side.

Arm action

Step 1	Bilateral inactive. The arms are held bilaterally, usually high and out to the side, although other positions behind or in front of the body may occur. Any arm action is usually slight and not consistent.
Step 2	Bilateral reactive. Arms swing upward briefly then are medially rotated at the shoulder in a winging movement prior to takeoff. It appears that this movement is in reaction to loss of balance.
Step 3	Bilateral assist. The arms pump up and down together, usually in front of the line of the trunk. Any downward and backward motion of the arms occurs after takeoff. The arms may move parallel to each other or be held at different levels as they move up and down.
Step 4	Semi-opposition. The arm on the side opposite the swing leg swings forward with that leg and back as the leg moves down. The position of the other arm is variable, often staying in front of the body or to the side.
Step 5	Opposing-assist. The arm opposite the swing leg moves forward and upward in synchrony with the forward and upward movement of that leg. The other arm moves in the direction opposite to the action of the swing leg. The range of movement in the arm action may be minimal unless the task requires speed or distance.

This sequence has been partially validated by Halverson and Williams (1985).

Reprinted, by permission, from M.A. Roberton and L.E. Halverson, 1984, *Developing Children—Their changing movement* (Philadelphia: Lea & Febiger), 56, 63.

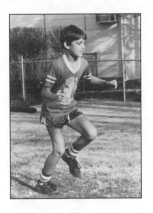
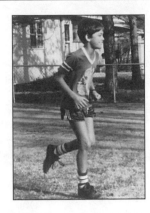
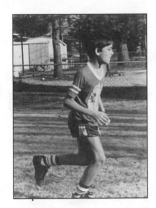

FIGURE 7.3   K.S., age 10.2 years, hopping.

OBSERVATION PLAN FOR HOPPING

LEG ACTION

Focus on the swing leg from the side. Is it active?

No — STEP 1 or 2
Focus on the support leg. Does it extend at takeoff to project the body upward?

Yes — STEP 3 or 4
Does the swing leg swing behind the support leg? Look at the support leg. Does the weight shift to the ball of the support foot before extension at takeoff?

No — STEP 1
Momentary flight

Yes — STEP 2
Fall and catch

No — STEP 3
Projected takeoff

Yes — STEP 1
Projection delay, swing leg leads

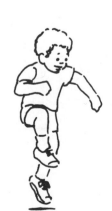
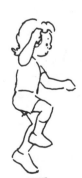
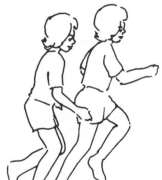
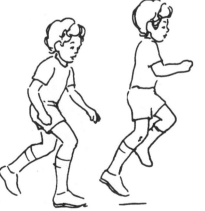

High, inactive swing leg
Support leg pulled up from floor
Step 1

Minimal extension at takeoff
Step 2

Takeoff leg is extending
Step 3

Swing leg leads
Swing leg is seen fully behind support leg
Support leg will fully extend at takeoff
Step 4

(continued)

(continued)

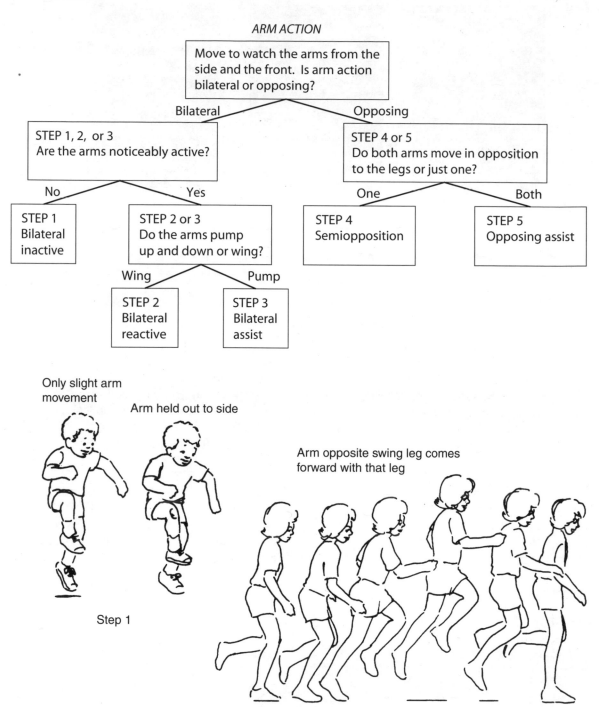

ARM ACTION

Move to watch the arms from the side and the front. Is arm action bilateral or opposing?

Bilateral — Opposing

STEP 1, 2, or 3
Are the arms noticeably active?

No — Yes

STEP 1
Bilateral inactive

STEP 2 or 3
Do the arms pump up and down or wing?

Wing — Pump

STEP 2
Bilateral reactive

STEP 3
Bilateral assist

STEP 4 or 5
Do both arms move in opposition to the legs or just one?

One — Both

STEP 4
Semiopposition

STEP 5
Opposing assist

Only slight arm movement

Arm held out to side

Arm opposite swing leg comes forward with that leg

Step 1

Step 4

Assessing the Developmental Level of Hopping

Observation Checklist: Hopping

Observation number	1	2	3	4	5	6	7
Hopper's name, photo, or video number							
Hopper's age, if known							
Date							
Observation type*							
Component							
Leg action							
Step 1 Momentary flight							
Step 2 Fall and catch; swing leg inactive							
Step 3 Projected takeoff; swing leg assists							
Step 4 Projection delay; swing leg leads							
Arm action							
Step 1 Bilateral inactive							
Step 2 Bilateral reactive							
Step 3 Bilateral assist							
Step 4 Semi-opposition							
Step 5 Opposing assist							
Summary profile							
Leg							
Arm							

*Codes for observation type: D = direct; P = photographs; F = film; V = video; S = slow motion.

From *Learning Activities for Life Span Motor Development Third Edition* by Kathleen Haywood and Nancy Getchell, 2001, Champaign, IL: Human Kinetics.

Reprinted, by permission, from M.A. Roberton and L.E. Halverson, 1984, *Developing Children—Their changing movement* (Philadelphia: Lea & Febiger), 54.

CHAPTER 8

Development of Ballistic Skills

Ballistic skills are those in which a person applies force to an object in order to project it. Throwing, kicking, and striking are all ballistic skills. It takes only a minute to think of many sports that involve one or more of these skills. So, proficient performance of ballistic skills is the key to participation in many common sport and recreation activities. An important skill for teachers, coaches, and therapists is accurate assessment of an individual's developmental level in throwing. Only by knowing someone's present developmental level can a teacher or coach know what learning and practice activities to plan or can a therapist know what therapeutic or conditioning program to design for that person.

The ballistic skills share many mechanical principles. This is especially true of those mechanical principles having to do with applying force to project an object. Expect developmental trends among the ballistic skills to overlap. Knowing the underlying mechanical principles involved is valuable because developmental sequences have not been validated for all the ballistic skills. The ballistic skill that has received the most attention is overarm throwing. You might want to make that your first observation activity so that you can use what you learn in observing other ballistic skills.

The ballistic skills typically occur very quickly, and there are several body components to observe. When categorizing performers it is helpful to have an observation plan. Plans are included for each activity in this chapter. Rather than comparing the list of developmental levels with a performance, you can make one decision at a time with an observation plan. The plan focuses your attention on an aspect of the movement pattern that will distinguish the developmental levels. With some performers, movement patterns are not "captured" by the observation plan. In this event you will have to refer to the more complete description in the developmental sequence table. More often, though, the plan will guide you to the appropriate developmental level for the performer under observation.

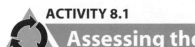

ACTIVITY 8.1

Assessing the Developmental Levels of Throwers

Purpose: To gain experience in assessing the developmental levels of throwers.

Throwing is probably the most common of the ballistic skills yet the most difficult to assess. This is true because of the number of body components to observe in addition to the backswing. To assess throwing, most of us must watch a person throw several balls, unless we videotape the thrower. In fact, at least one categorization cannot be done with the naked eye, so working from sequential still photographs, slow motion videotapes, or video clips is a good way to learn the assessment process and to categorize throwers.

To categorize throwers you should use the Developmental Sequence for Throwing (see table 8.1 on pp. 101-102) for the trunk, backswing, humerus (upper arm), forearm, and feet, as well as the observation plan (pp. 103-106). Carefully study the developmental sequence before your observation; then use the observation plan as you observe the thrower directly or on video. The checklist gives a brief title for each developmental step. Once you have worked your way through the decisions in the observation plan and arrived at a developmental step, or level, place a check mark on the checklist (record sheet 8.1 on pp. 107-108) corresponding to that level. Remember that the observation plan is necessarily brief and that the developmental sequence table provides more detail to cover the range of movements you are likely to observe.

Table 8.1 describes four developmental steps for foot action. The observation plan directs you to watch the thrower from the side and note whether a step is taken. If not, the thrower is in Step 1; if so, you need to observe which leg (homo-, same side; or contralateral, opposite side) is stepping. If it is the homolateral leg, the thrower is in Step 2. If it is the contralateral leg, you are to observe the length of the step. If the step length is less than half the thrower's height, the thrower is in Step 3; but if it is greater, the thrower is in Step 4. The observation plan next directs you to watch the trunk during a throw. Table 8.1 describes three levels of trunk action. The observation plan focuses your attention on whether or not the trunk rotates. If not, the thrower is in Step 1; if so, you are to observe whether the hips rotate before the upper trunk. If not, the thrower is in Step 2. If the hips rotate first, the thrower is in Step 3.

The next component in the observation plan is the backswing. Table 8.1 describes four steps for the backswing. The observation plan directs you to watch for the arm moving backward before the throw. If it does not, the thrower is in Step 1. If it does, you should watch to see if the hand drops below the waist. If not, the thrower is in Step 2 or 3. If the backward movement is by arm flexion on the trunk, the thrower is in Step 2; but if the backward movement is circular, out and around, the thrower is in Step 3. If the thrower drops the hand below the waist and continues in a circular, downward backswing, the thrower is in Step 4.

Finally, watch the action of the upper arm, or humerus, and then the forearm. The table describes three levels of each. The observation plan calls for you to watch from the side. If the upper arm does not swing forward at shoulder level, that is, if it is either angled down or angled up, the thrower is in Step 1. If the upper arm swings at shoulder level, you must watch to see if the elbow comes forward ahead of the trunk, or if the elbow lags behind and you can see it in the outline of the trunk as the trunk swings around to "front-facing." In the first case, the thrower is in Step 2; in the second case, he/she is in Step 3. As you observe the forearm, you must watch to see if it moves steadily forward with the throw, indicating that the thrower is Step 1, or whether it drops downward/stays stationary as the thrower rotates the trunk forward. If it drops down or remains stationary, look to see whether the deepest drop (or lag) is before the trunk reaches front-facing (Step 2) or is at front-facing (Step 3). This latter distinction can be difficult or impossible to see without slow motion video.

Equipment List

Tennis ball

Cones or tape for marking a restraining line

Instructions

1. In this activity you will categorize throwers for their developmental levels of throwing. Use the Developmental Sequence for Throwing (table 8.1) and the observation plan to guide your decisions. First, categorize the thrower shown in the sequential still photos of figure 8.1 on page 102.

2. Next, open your CD-ROM, and select the folder labeled Chapter 8 and then the folder labeled Throwing. Work through the two examples in Set A. The program will prompt you to watch for the critical elements, just as the observation plan does.

3. After completing Set A, categorize examples in Set B as indicated by your instructor. Label a column on record sheet 8.1 (pp. 107-108) for each video example. You will have to follow the observation plan (pp. 103-106) yourself with the Set B videos. As you arrive at a developmental level for each component, check that level in the appropriate column on record sheet 8.1.

4. After categorizing the photos and videos, arrange to categorize a child directly. When categorizing throwers pictured in drawings, photos, or videos, all you can assume is that the thrower has been instructed to throw for distance. When doing direct observations, you are responsible for giving throwers instructions. Direct your throwers to throw as far as possible without hurting their arms. You might want to indicate a restraining line and tell throwers they can run up to the line but should release the ball before crossing it. Unless you are observing small children, you should conduct your observation outside in a large space.

5. In live observations and when throwers use movements at different levels from throw to throw, the practice is to place them at the level you observe most often. For example, if out of five turns the thrower is Step 2 in three turns and Step 3 in two turns, place the thrower at Step 2.

Questions

1. Did throwers tend to be at the same step number for each of the body components, for example, Step 2, or did they tend to be at different steps for different body components? Cite an example from your checklist.

2. Among the throwers you observed, was there an older child or adult at a lower level in some body component than a younger thrower? Describe any such occurrence.

3. On your direct observations of a thrower, did you notice whether he or she or she used movements characteristic of different levels from throw to throw? If so, describe this situation.

4. Consider the range of individual functional and structural constraints. Name an individual, structural constraint that, if changed, would alter the movement pattern of the thrower. Indicate the body component(s) that would change and how it (they) would change.

5. Consider task and environmental constraints. Choose a constraint that, if changed, would change the movement pattern of the thrower. Indicate the body component(s) that would change and how it (they) would change.

6. Which method of observation (photos, videos, direct) did you find the easiest? Which did you find the hardest? Why? What are the advantages and disadvantages of each?

TABLE 8.1

Developmental Sequence for Throwing

Trunk action in throwing and striking for force

Step 1	No trunk action or forward-backward movements. Only the arm is active in force production. Sometimes the forward thrust of the arm pulls the trunk into a passive left rotation (assuming a right-handed throw), but no twist-up precedes that action. If trunk action occurs, it accompanies the forward thrust of the arm by flexing forward at the hips. Preparatory extension sometimes precedes forward hip flexion.
Step 2	Upper trunk rotation or total trunk "block" rotation. The spine and pelvis rotate away from the intended line of flight and then simultaneously begin forward rotation, acting as a unit, or "block." Occasionally, only the upper spine twists away, then toward the direction of force. The pelvis, then, remains fixed, facing the line of flight, or joins the rotary movement after forward spinal rotation has begun.
Step 3	Differentiated rotation. The pelvis precedes the upper spine in initiating forward rotation. The child twists away from the intended line of ball flight and then begins forward rotation with the pelvis while the upper spine is still twisting away.

Backswing, humerus, and forearm action in the overarm throw for force

Preparatory arm backswing component

Step 1	No backswing. The ball in the hand moves directly forward to release from the arm's original position when the hand first grasped the ball.
Step 2	Elbow and humeral flexion. The ball moves away from the intended line of flight to a position behind or alongside the head by upward flexion of the humerus and concomitant elbow flexion.
Step 3	Circular, upward backswing. The ball moves away from the intended line of flight to a position behind the head via a circular overhead movement with elbow extended, or an oblique swing back, or a vertical lift from the hip.
Step 4	Circular, downward backswing. The ball moves away from the intended line of flight to a position behind the head via a circular, down-and-back motion, which carries the hand below the waist.

Humerus (upper arm) action component during forward swing

Step 1	Humerus oblique. The upper arm moves forward to ball release in a plane that intersects the trunk obliquely above or below the horizontal line of the shoulders. Occasionally, during the backswing, the upper arm is placed at a right angle to the trunk, with the elbow pointing toward the target. It maintains this fixed position during the throw.
Step 2	Humerus aligned but independent. The upper arm moves forward to ball release in a plane horizontally aligned with the shoulder, forming a right angle between humerus and trunk. By the time the shoulders (upper spine) reach front-facing, the upper arm and elbow have moved independently ahead of the outline of the body (as seen from the side) via horizontal adduction at the shoulder.

(continued)

TABLE 8.1 *(continued)*

Step 3	Humerus lags. The upper arm moves forward to ball release horizontally aligned, but at the moment the shoulders (upper spine) reach front-facing, the upper arm remains within the outline of the body (as seen from the side). No horizontal adduction of the upper arm occurs before front-facing.

Forearm action component during forward swing

Step 1	No forearm lag. The forearm and ball move steadily forward to ball release throughout the throwing action.
Step 2	Forearm lag. The forearm and ball appear to lag, that is, to remain stationary behind the child or to move downward or backward in relation to the child. The lagging forearm reaches its farthest point back, deepest point down, or last stationary point before the shoulders (upper spine) reach front-facing.
Step 3	Delayed forearm lag. The lagging forearm delays reaching its final point of lag until the moment of front-facing.

Action of the feet in forceful throwing and striking

Step 1	No step. The child throws from the initial foot position.
Step 2	Homolateral step. The child steps with the foot on the same side as the throwing hand.
Step 3	Contralateral, short step. The child steps with the foot on the opposite side from the throwing hand.
Step 4	Contralateral, long step. The child steps with the opposite foot a distance of over half the child's standing height.

Validation studies support the trunk sequence (Roberton, 1977; Roberton, 1978a; Roberton & Langendorfer, 1980; Langendorfer, 1982; Roberton & DiRocco, 1981.) Validation studies support the arm sequences for the overarm throw (Halverson, Roberton, & Langendorfer, 1982; Roberton, 1977; Roberton, 1978a; Roberton & Langendorfer, 1980; Roberton & DiRocco, 1981) with the exception of the preparatory arm backswing sequence, which was hypothesized by Roberton (1984) from the work of Langendorfer (1980). Langendorfer (1982) believes the humerus and forearm components are appropriate for overarm striking. The foot action sequence was hypothesized by Roberton (1984) from the work of Leme and Shambes (1978); Seefeldt, Reuschlein, and Vogel (1972); and Wild (1937).

Reprinted, by permission, from M.A. Roberton and L.E. Halverson, 1984, *Developing children—Their changing movement* (Philadelphia: Lea & Febiger), 103, 106-107, 118.

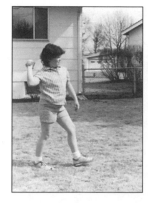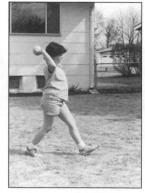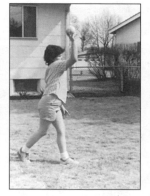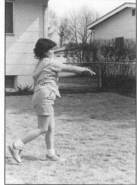

FIGURE 8.1   C.H., age 8.9 years, throwing.

OBSERVATION PLAN FOR THROWING

FOOT ACTION

Watch the feet from the side. Is a step taken?

— No → **STEP 1** No step

— Yes → **STEP 2, 3, or 4** Is the step homo- or contralateral?

— Homo- → **STEP 2** Homolateral step

— Contra- → **STEP 3** Is the step over half the thrower's height?

— No → **STEP 3** Contralateral, short step

— Yes → **STEP 4** Contralateral, long step

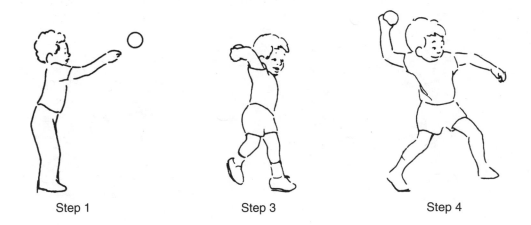

Step 1   Step 3   Step 4

(continued)

(continued)

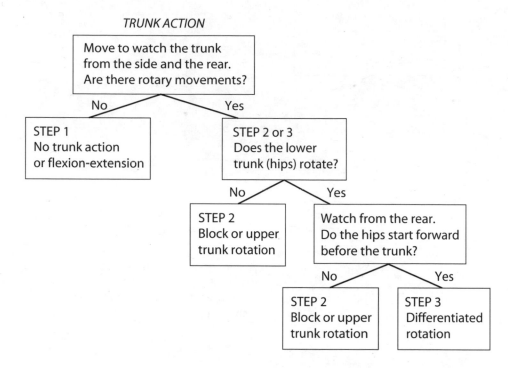

TRUNK ACTION

Move to watch the trunk from the side and the rear. Are there rotary movements?

No → STEP 1
No trunk action or flexion-extension

Yes → STEP 2 or 3
Does the lower trunk (hips) rotate?

No → STEP 2
Block or upper trunk rotation

Yes → Watch from the rear. Do the hips start forward before the trunk?

No → STEP 2
Block or upper trunk rotation

Yes → STEP 3
Differentiated rotation

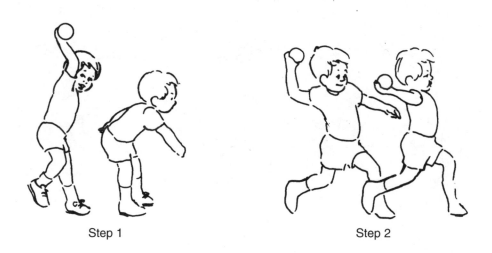

Step 1   Step 2

BACKSWING

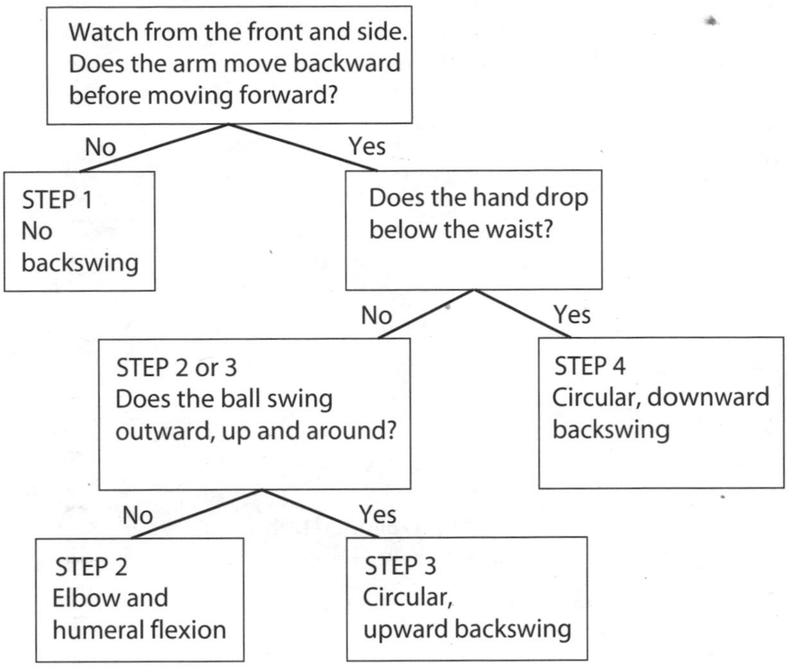

Watch from the front and side.
Does the arm move backward
before moving forward?

No — Yes

STEP 1
No
backswing

Does the hand drop
below the waist?

No — Yes

STEP 2 or 3
Does the ball swing
outward, up and around?

STEP 4
Circular, downward
backswing

No — Yes

STEP 2
Elbow and
humeral flexion

STEP 3
Circular,
upward backswing

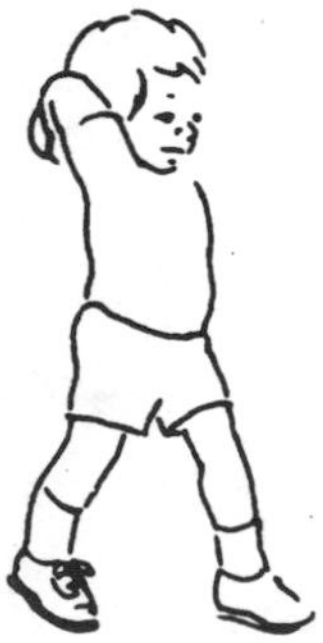

Step 2

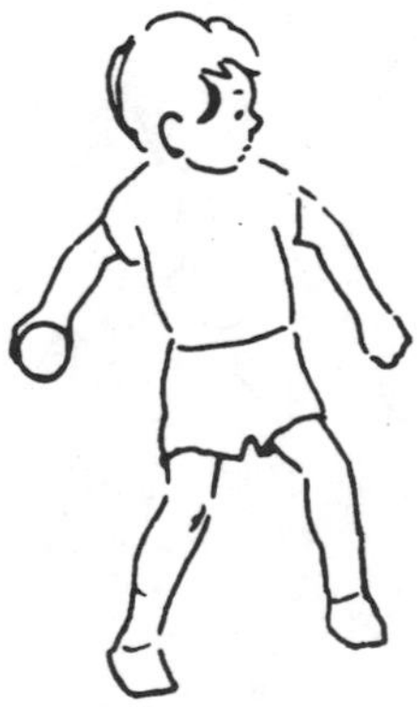

Step 4

(continued)

(continued)

HUMERUS ACTION

Watch from the side. Do the elbow and upper arm move forward at shoulder level (humerus forms a right angle with the trunk)?

No → STEP 1 Humerus oblique

Yes → STEP 2 or 3 At the moment of front-facing, is the elbow pointed toward you at the side, or is it seen outside the outline of the body?

Outside → STEP 2 Humerus aligned but independent

To side → STEP 3 Humerus lags

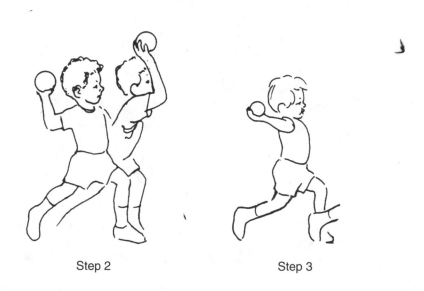

Step 2   Step 3

FOREARM

Watch the ball in the thrower's hand. Does it move forward steadily or drop downward or stay stationary as the thrower rotates forward?

Steadily forward → STEP 1 No forearm lag

Drops down/stays stationary → Is the deepest lag reached before or at front-facing? (May be difficult to see without slow-motion film or videot...

Before → STEP 2 Forearm lag

At → STEP 3 Delayed forearm lag

ACTIVITY 8.2

Assessing the Developmental Levels of Strikers

Purpose: To gain experience in assessing the developmental levels of strikers.

There are many forms of striking. The striking motion can be made overhead, sidearm, or underarm (as in the golf swing). Contact with the object can be with the hand or with an implement, and the implement can have a short or long handle. The striking tasks in sports must sometimes conform to rules. Such rules might govern the striking implement, the position of the striker, and the striker's movement—for example, staying behind a restraining line.

All of the ballistic skills share many principles of stability and motion. This is particularly true of the striking skills. In this learning activity you will observe sidearm striking, but keep in mind that you can adapt the tools used here to observe other types of striking. In fact, the foot action, trunk action, and upper arm action sequences are the same as for throwing.

In the previous activity, we described the use of the developmental sequence table for throwing, the Observation Plan for Throwing, and the observation checklist. Similar tools are provided here and are used in the same way. If you did not complete activity 8.1, read the introduction to activity 8.1 and use the Developmental Sequence for Sidearm Striking (table 8.2 on p. 110), the Observation Plan for Sidearm Striking (pp. 111-112), and record sheet 8.2 (pp. 113-1￼) in the same manner. Note that the foot, trunk, and upper arm actions are actual'￼ ￼en from the throwing sequence and observation plan.

Equipment List

Tennis ball

Racket of appropriate size for the selected individual

Instructions

1. In this activity you will categorize sidearm strikers for their developmental levels of striking. Use the Developmental Sequence for Sidearm Striking (table 8.2) and the observation plan (pp. 111-112) to guide your decisions. First, categorize the striker shown in the sequential still photos of figure 8.2 on page 111. Record your decisions on record sheet 8.2 (pp. 113-114).

2. Next, open your CD-ROM; select the folder labeled Chapter 8 and then the folder labeled Striking. Work through the two examples in Set A. The program will prompt you to watch for the critical elements, just as in the observation plan.

3. After completing Set A, categorize examples in Set B as directed by your instructor. Label a column on record sheet 8.2 for each video example. You will have to follow the observation plan yourself on the Set B examples. As you arrive at a developmental level for each component, check that level in the appropriate column on the record sheet.

4. After categorizing the photos and videos, arrange to categorize a child or youth directly. It is ideal to work in pairs so that one person can toss the ball underhanded to the striker while the other person observes the striker's movements. When doing direct observations, instruct your strikers to "hit the ball hard." Although strikers at the more advanced levels stand sideways, do not give any directions about the direction to face. Make this part of your observation. If your striker performs at different levels from attempt to attempt, assign the developmental level you observe most often (the modal level).

Questions

1. Did the strikers tend to be at the same step number for each of the body components, for example, Step 2, or did they tend to be at different steps for different body components? Cite an example from your checklist.

2. Among the group of strikers you observed, was there an older child or adult at a lower level than a younger striker in some body component? Describe any such occurrence.

3. On your direct observations of a striker, did you notice if your striker used movements characteristic of different levels from turn to turn? If so, describe this situation.

4. Consider the racket you provided. How did the racket constrain the movement pattern of the striker? If you observed a range of ages and sizes of strikers, what could you change (or scale) about the racket to afford some of the strikers a different movement? (For example, the racket may have been too long for a short child.) How do you think this would change the movement?

TABLE 8.2

Developmental Sequence for Sidearm Striking
Racket action component
Step 1   Chop. The racket is swung in the vertical plane.
Step 2   Arm swing only. The racket swings ahead of the trunk.
Step 3   Racket lag. The racket lags behind trunk rotation but goes ahead of the trunk at front-facing.
Step 4   Delayed racket lag. The racket is still lagging behind the trunk at front-facing.
Foot, trunk, and upper arm action component
See the foot, trunk, and upper arm sections in table 8.1.

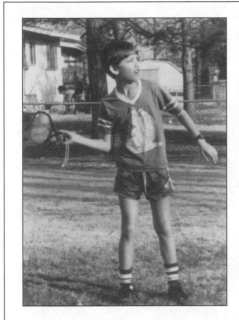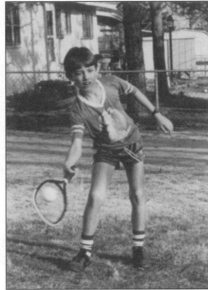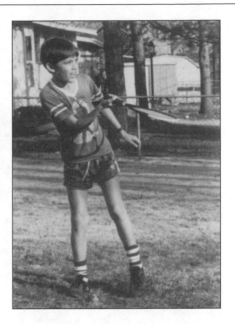

FIGURE 8.2 K.S., age 10.2 years, striking.

OBSERVATION PLAN FOR SIDEARM STRIKING
(for foot, trunk and humerus components, use the throwing observation)

RACKET/BAT ACTION

Is the racket swung in a horizontal plane?

No → STEP 1 Chop

Yes → STEP 2 to 4 Does the racket "lag" (pause in forward motion)?

No → STEP 2 Arm swing only

Yes → Does the racket "lag" occur at the front-facing position?

No → STEP 3 Racket lag

Yes → STEP 4 Delayed racket lag

(continued)

111

(continued)

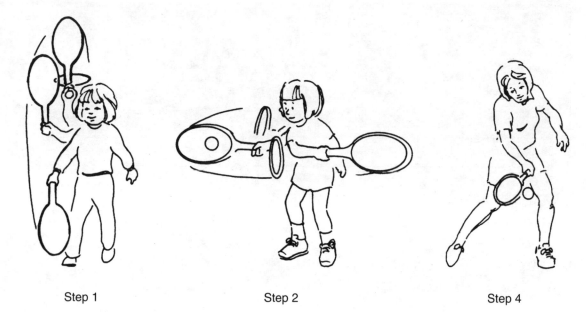

Step 1   Step 2   Step 4

Assessing the Developmental Level of Sidearm Striking

Observation Checklist: Striking

Observation number	1	2	3	4	5	6	7
Striker's name, photo, or video number							
Striker's age, if known							
Date							
Observation type*							
Component							
Racket/bat action							
Step 1 Chop							
Step 2 Arm swing only							
Step 3 Racket Lag							
Step 4 Delayed Lag							
Humerus action							
Step 1 Humerus oblique							
Step 2 Aligned, independent							
Step 3 Humerus lags							
Trunk action							
Step 1 None/forward-back							
Step 2 Block/upper trunk							
Step 3 Differentiated rotation							
Foot action							
Step 1 No step							
Step 2 Homolateral							
Step 3 Contralateral, short							
Step 4 Contralateral, long							

*Codes for observation type: D = direct; P = photographs; F = film; V = video; S = slow motion.

(continued)

From *Learning Activities for Life Span Motor Development Third Edition* by Kathleen Haywood and Nancy Getchell, 2001, Champaign, IL: Human Kinetics.

Observation number	1	2	3	4	5	6	7
Summary profile							
Racket							
Humerus							
Trunk							
Foot							

*Codes for observation type: D = direct; P = photographs; F = film; V = video; S = slow motion.

From *Learning Activities for Life Span Motor Development Third Edition* by Kathleen Haywood and Nancy Getchell, 2001, Champaign, IL: Human Kinetics.

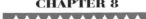

ACTIVITY 8.3

Assessing the Developmental Levels of Punters

Purpose: To gain experience in assessing the developmental levels of punters.

Both kicking and punting involve striking a ball with the foot. In punting, though, the ball is dropped from the hands. We have acknowledged that the ballistic skills share many principles of stability and motion. You will notice similarities between the leg action of kicking/punting and the arm action in throwing. The trunk and leg actions among kicking/punting, throwing, and striking also are similar.

In this activity you will assess the developmental level of punters. In contrast to kicking, a developmental sequence for punting has been hypothesized from longitudinal observations of children. This sequence has not been validated (that is, tested to see whether it meets the criteria for stage-wise progression), but is useful in distinguishing punters of different developmental levels.

In activity 8.1, we described use of the developmental sequence table for throwing, the Observation Plan for Throwing, and the observation checklist. Similar tools are provided here for punting and are used in the same way. If you did not complete activity 8.1, read the introduction to activity 8.1 (p. 99) and use the Developmental Sequence for Punting (table 8.3), the Observation Plan for Punting (pp. 117-119), and record sheet 8.3 (p. 120). You should use the observation checklist for punting in the same manner as described for throwing.

Equipment List

Playground ball (or other soft ball for young children)

Instructions

1. In this activity you will categorize punters for their developmental levels of punting. Use the Developmental Sequence for Punting (table 8.3) and the observation plan (pp. 117-119) to guide your decisions. Open your CD-ROM; select the folder labeled Chapter 8 and then the folder labeled Punting. Work through the two examples in Set A. The program will prompt you to watch for the critical elements, just as the observation plan does.

2. After completing Set A, categorize examples in Set B as directed by your instructor. Label a column on record sheet 8.3 (p. 120) for each video example. You will have to follow the observation plan yourself for the Set B examples. As you arrive at a developmental level for each component, check that level in the appropriate column on record sheet 8.3.

3. After categorizing the videos, arrange to categorize a child or youth directly. When categorizing punters pictured in drawings, photos, or videos, you must assume that the punter has been instructed to punt for distance. When doing direct observations, you are responsible for giving punters instructions. Direct your punters to punt as far as possible. Unless you are observing small children, you should conduct your observation outside in a large space.

4. In live observations and when punters use movements at different levels from punt to punt, the practice is to place them at the level you observe most often (the modal level). For example, out of five turns if the punter is at Step 2 three times and at Step 3 two times, place the punter at Step 2).

Questions

1. Did punters tend to be at the same step number for each of the body components, for example, Step 2, or did they tend to be at different steps for different body components? Cite an example from your checklist.

2. Among the group of punters you observed, was there an older child or adult at a lower level than a younger punter in some body component? Describe any such occurrence.

3. On your direct observations of a punter, did you notice if your punter used movements characteristic of different levels from punt to punt? If so, describe this situation.

4. Consider the range of individual functional and structural constraints. Name an individual, structural constraint that, if changed, would alter the movement pattern of the punter. Indicate the body component(s) of the developmental sequence that would change and how it (they) would change.

5. Consider task and environmental constraints. Choose a constraint that, if modified, would change the movement pattern of the punter. Indicate the body component(s) that would change and how it (they) would change.

6. Which method of observation (videos or direct) did you find the easiest? Which did you find the hardest? Why? What are the advantages and disadvantages of each?

TABLE 8.3

Developmental Sequence for Punting

Ball-release phase: arm component

Step 1	Upward toss. Hands are on the sides of the ball. The ball is tossed upward from both hands after the support foot has landed (if a step was taken).
Step 2	Late drop from chest height. Hands hard on the sides of the ball. The ball is dropped from chest height after the support foot has landed (if a step was taken).
Step 3	Late drop from waist height. Hands are on the sides of the ball. The ball is lifted upward and forward from waist level. It is released at the same time as, or just prior to, the landing of the support foot.
Step 4	Early drop from chest height. One hand is rotated to the side and under the ball. The other hand is rotated to the side and top of the ball. The hands carry the ball on a forward and upward path during the approach. The ball is released at chest level as the final approach stride begins.

Ball-contact phase: arm component

Step 1	Arms drop. Arms drop bilaterally from ball release to a position on each side of the hips at ball contact.
Step 2	Arms abduct. Arms bilaterally abduct after ball release. The arm on the side of the kicking leg may pull back as that leg swings forward.
Step 3	Arm opposition. After ball release, the arms bilaterally abduct during flight. At contact, the arm opposite the kicking leg has swung forward with that leg. The arm on the side of the kicking leg remains abducted and to the rear.

Ball-contact phase: leg action component	
Step 1	No/short step; ankle flexed. No step or one short step is taken. The kicking leg swings forward from a position parallel to or slightly behind the support foot. The knee may be totally extended by contact or, more frequently, still flexed 90° with contact above or below the knee joint. The thigh is still moving upward at contact. The ankle tends to be (dorsi-)flexed.
Step 2	Long step; ankle extension. Several steps may be taken. The last step onto the support leg is a long stride. The thigh of the kicking leg has slowed or stopped forward motion at contact. The ankle is extended (plantarflexed). The knee has 20° to 30° of extension still possible by contact [knee is not completely extended].
Step 3	Leap and hop. The individual may take several steps, but the last is actually a leap onto the support foot. After contact, the momentum of the kicking leg pulls the individual off the ground in a hop.

This sequence was hypothesized by Roberton (1984) and has not been validated.

Reprinted, by permission, from M.A. Roberton and L.E. Halverson, 1984, *Developing children—Their changing movement* (Philadelphia: Lea & Febiger), 123.

OBSERVATION PLAN FOR PUNTING

BALL-RELEASE PHASE: ARM ACTION

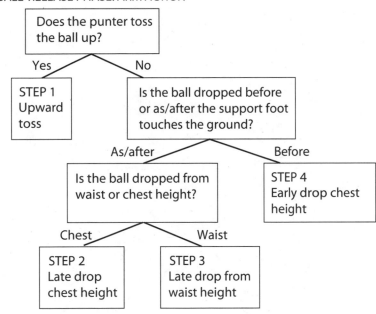

(continued)

(continued)

BALL-CONTACT PHASE: ARM COMPONENT

Do the arms drop to
the sides after ball release?

Yes   No

STEP 1
Arms drop

Do the arms move together
out to the side after release
or do they move in opposition?

Side   Opposition

STEP 2
Arms abduct

STEP 3
Arms opposition

Arm action,
Step 4

Arm component,
Step 1

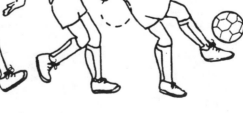

Arm component,
Step 3

Line art drawn from film tracings from the Motor Development and Child Study Laboratory, University of Wisconsin–Madison.

BALL-CONTACT PHASE: LEG ACTION COMPONENT

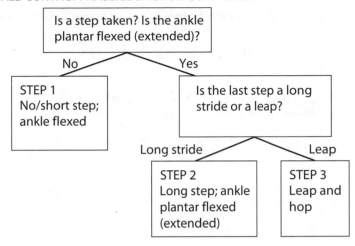

Is a step taken? Is the ankle plantar flexed (extended)?

No → STEP 1
No/short step; ankle flexed

Yes → Is the last step a long stride or a leap?

Long stride → STEP 2
Long step; ankle plantar flexed (extended)

Leap → STEP 3
Leap and hop

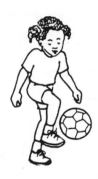

Leg action component,
Step 1

Line art drawn from film tracings from the Motor Development and Child Study Laboratory, University of Wisconsin–Madison.

Assessing the Developmental Level of Punting

Observation Checklist: Punting

Observation number	1	2	3	4	5	6	7
Punter's name, photo, or video number							
Punter's age, if known							
Date							
Observation type*							
Component							
Ball-release phase: arm							
Step 1 Upward toss							
Step 2 Late drop from chest height							
Step 3 Late drop from waist height							
Step 4 Early drop from chest height							
Ball-contact phase: arm							
Step 1 Arms drop							
Step 2 Arms abduct							
Step 3 Arm opposition							
Ball-contact phase: leg							
Step 1 No/short step; ankle flexed							
Step 2 Long step; ankle extension							
Step 3 Leap and hop							
Summary profile							
Ball release: arm							
Ball contact: arm							
Ball contact: leg							

*Codes for observation type: D = direct; P = photographs; F = film; V = video; S = slow motion.

From *Learning Activities for Life Span Motor Development Third Edition* by Kathleen Haywood and Nancy Getchell, 2001, Champaign, IL: Human Kinetics.

ACTIVITY 8.4

Comparing Throws for Force With Throws for Accuracy

Purpose: To observe changes in movement patterns by switching a task constraint from the goal of force to the goal of accuracy.

Just as changing an individual or environmental constraint can affect the movement arising from the interaction of constraints, so can changing the task constraint. Here, we will observe changes in the movement pattern as the task goal is switched from force to accuracy. Researchers have examined this very issue. Langendorfer (1990) observed 9- to 10-year-olds and adults throwing for distance and accuracy. He found that especially male throwers used the movement patterns characteristic of lower developmental steps when throwing for accuracy compared to distance. Williams, Haywood, and VanSant (1993, 1996) observed the same situation with older adults. The older adult throwers demonstrated a slower throwing velocity in the accuracy condition than in the distance condition.

The issue of changing movement patterns with a change in the goal of the task is an important one for teachers, coaches, and therapists. If, indeed, movement patterns change with the goal, instructors must be clear in giving directions as to the goal of a task. This is particularly true when the instructor would like to assess the performer at his or her best, that is, undertaking an optimal effort. This issue also is important with regard to planning instructional or therapeutic activities. If some goals elicit certain movement patterns and other goals other movement patterns, an instructor sometimes can elicit a different movement pattern from a performer by changing the goal of the task.

In this activity, you will use Langendorfer's method to compare performers throwing for distance and then for accuracy.

Equipment List

Tennis ball

Tape to mark an 8 ft (2.4 m) circular target on a gymnasium wall

Tape to mark 6.5 yd and 11 yd (6 m and 10 m) restraining lines on the floor

Instructions

1. Locate three individuals of different ages to be throwers in this observation. Each of the throwers should make seven throws for distance, that is, throwing as far as possible. If you are able to videotape the thrower, you need only videotape three throws. For throwers other than small children, the observation should be conducted on a large field. In your instructions to throwers, emphasize that they should throw as far as possible without hurting themselves.

2. Using the same type of ball, each thrower should make seven throws (three videotaped throws) at a target. As nearly as possible, use the environment in the study by Langendorfer (1990): an 8 ft (2.4 m) circular target and a throwing distance of 11 yd (10 m) for adults and 6.5 yd (6 m) for children. In your instructions to throwers, emphasize hitting the target.

3. For all throws, use the Developmental Sequence for Throwing (table 8.1 on pp. 101-102) and the Observation Plan for Throwing (pp. 103-106) to place the throwers in developmental levels for each component.

4. On record sheet 8.4, label two columns for each thrower, one for each of the two conditions (force and accuracy). For this activity, you are observing the movement pattern and need not be concerned with the distance of the distance throws or the accuracy of the accuracy throws.

Questions

1. Compare the summary profiles for distance versus accuracy throws for each of your three throwers. Are they different? If so, how are they different?

2. Aside from the developmental levels, did you notice other differences when your performers were throwing for distance versus accuracy? What were they?

3. Did the age of your throwers make a difference in the extent of change, if any, between the distance and the accuracy condition? If so, how?

4. Were the conditions you provided (the area, the ball, the size of the target, the throwing distance for accuracy) reasonable for all your throwers? If not, why not, and what would you change if you were to repeat this observation?

5. Identify other skills that would also be affected by a change in the goal of the task. Indicate how the movement patterns for these skills would change.

Assessing the Developmental Level of Throwing

Observation Checklist: Throwing

Observation number	1	2	3	4	5	6	7
Thrower's name, photo, or video number							
Thrower's age, if known							
Date							
Force or accuracy?							
Component							
Foot action							
Step 1 No step							
Step 2 Homolateral							
Step 3 Contralateral, short							
Step 4 Contralateral, long							
Trunk action							
Step 1 None/forward-back							
Step 2 Block/upper trunk only							
Step 3 Differentiated rotation							
Arm action: backswing							
Step 1 No backswing							
Step 2 Elbow and humeral flexion							
Step 3 Circular, upward							
Step 4 Circular, downward							
Arm action: humerus							
Step 1 Humerus oblique							
Step 2 Humerus aligned, independent							
Step 3 Humerus lags							

From *Learning Activities for Life Span Motor Development Third Edition* by Kathleen Haywood and Nancy Getchell, 2001, Champaign, IL: Human Kinetics.

(continued)

Observation number	1	2	3	4	5	6	7
Component							
Arm action: forearm							
Step 1 No lag							
Step 2 Forearm lag							
Step 3 Delayed lag							
Summary profile							
Foot							
Trunk							
Backswing							
Humerus							
Forearm							

From *Learning Activities for Life Span Motor Development Third Edition* by Kathleen Haywood and Nancy Getchell, 2001, Champaign, IL: Human Kinetics.

CHAPTER 9

Development of Manipulative Skills

Many animals have locomotor skills. Some can even travel faster than humans. No life-form, though, can match humans in manual dexterity. Humans can perform a wide range of skills with the hands—from the tiniest, most intricate movements to large movements with large objects. As developmentalists, we are interested in the full range of manipulative skills that humans perform. We are interested in reaching and grasping and their development. We also are interested in sport skills that involve manipulation, especially catching—probably the most common manipulative sport skill.

As with the other groups of fundamental skills, the manipulative skills share certain mechanical principles. The chief principle underlying the manipulative sport skills is that "giving" with the arms or implement intercepting an object allows force to be dissipated over distance and time. Hence force is absorbed in such a way that the object can be retained and controlled.

In this chapter, you will have the opportunity to observe grasping development in infants as well as the opportunity to assess catching development in children. To assess catching we use tools similar to those we used for the locomotor and ballistic skills: a developmental sequence organized by body component, an observation plan, and a checklist based on the developmental sequence. At the end of the chapter you will have an opportunity to hypothesize your own developmental sequence for a skill of your (or your instructor's) choice. This is a tool you can use numerous times for many skills to conduct assessments when a researched and published developmental sequence is not available.

ACTIVITY 9.1

Observing Grasping Development

Purpose: To observe the types of grips an infant uses to grasp objects of varying shape and size.

One of the earliest-developing manipulative skills is grasping. A grasp is typically the culmination of an arm reach for an object. In the 1930s, H.M. Halverson studied the development of grasping in infants 16 to 52 weeks of age. He observed 10 stages of grasping development describing the grip configuration used at each stage (see table 9.1 on p. 128). The grip configurations used in the early stages of grasping development are collectively·called power grips because the object is held against the palm of the hand. The grip configurations in the later stages are called precision grips because objects are held between the thumb and one or more of the fingers. The infants observed by Halverson made the transition from power grips to precision grips at about 9 months of age.

Halverson held the environmental and task constraints in his observation constant. Of particular note is that the object grasped was always a 1 in. (2.5 cm) cube. More recently, as researchers came to view movement as arising from the interaction of constraints, they replicated Halverson's work with objects of varying shape and size. Although they still observed the transition from power to precision grips, the age at which infants used specific types of grips varied with the size and shape of the object.

We now understand that explaining grasping development is more complicated than saying that an infant is "x" months old so he or she will use grip "y." Infants of a given age can use a variety of grips depending on the size and shape of the object. For example, an infant might use a power grip to grasp a block that is large compared to the infant's hand size but a precision grip to grasp a small block. In this observation we will see how an infant changes the grip as the object to be picked up changes. We will see how the grips used and the infant's age compare to the developmental stages Halverson published in 1931.

Equipment List

Infant high chair (with chair and tray or table)

Two to three building blocks of different sizes

Three small objects that vary in size, weight, and shape but are small enough for an infant to pick up with one hand (small plastic cup, rattle, small ball, etc.)

Instructions

1. Select an infant between 6 and 12 months of age. Position the infant sitting upright in front of a table or tray such that he or she could easily pick up an object from the surface (the infant can be held). For this observation, do not vary the infant's position or the distance from the table or tray. Only the size and shape of the object are to be varied. If possible, observe the infant during a time period when the infant is rested and playful.

2. One by one, place each of the objects directly in front of the infant and observe the grip used by the infant to pick it up. You might have to tap on the table to get the infant to focus on the object. If any of the objects is small enough to be swallowed, you are responsible for monitoring the infant's play with the object. Do not allow the infant to place the small object in his or her mouth.

3. Use table 9.1 to determine which grip, as originally described by Halverson, the infant used. (With the parents' permission you can videotape the infant and make this determination later from the videotape.) Record this information on record sheet 9.1 on page 129.

4. If you have time and the infant is attentive, place each of the objects in front of the infant a second time and determine the grip used; observe whether the same grip is used for the same object both times.

Questions

1. How many different grips did the infant use in your observation session?

2. How does your infant's age compare to the age ranges Halverson published for the grips that your infant used?

3. What trends did you notice in the type of grip the infant used to pick up the various objects? For example, was there a particular object size or weight that when exceeded resulted in the infant's using a power grip rather than a precision grip? Explain. Note: Grips 3 through 7 in Halverson's sequence are power grips whereas 8, 9, and 10 are precision grips.

4. Were there particular shapes that resulted in the infant's using a power grip or precision grip? Explain.

5. Did you notice any times the infant attempted to pick up the object, dropped it, and then grasped it again using a different grip configuration? Explain which grips were used and identify the size, shape, and weight of the object.

6. Did the infant change the grip used on any of the second offerings? Which ones? Why do you think this was so?

TABLE 9.1

Observation Scale for Grasping Development

Type of grasp	Average age (months)	Age range (months)
1. Makes no contact with block	4.0	4.0-8.0
2. Makes contact with block but does not secure it	5.0	4.0-13.0
3. Primitive squeeze: Thrusts hand beyond block, then pulls it toward self until squeezed against body or other hand	5.0	5.0-6.0
4. Squeeze grasp: Hand approaches from side, fingers close on block to press it against heel of palm; cannot raise block	6.0	5.0-8.0
5. Hand grasp: Hand is brought down on block, and block is squeezed against heel of palm with fingers on far side, thumb on adjacent side	7.0	5.0-13.0
6. Palm grasp: Hand is brought down on block as above, but thumb is placed on near surface to oppose the fingers	7.0	5.0-10.0
7. Superior palm: Thumb side of the hand is brought down on the block with the thumb on near side and the first two fingers on the far side	8.0	7.0-13.0
8. Inferior forefinger: As above [in #7] but block is not held against palm; grasp maintained with fingers	9.0	8.0-13.0
9. Forefinger: Block is grasped with fingertips, thumb opposing first two or three fingers	13.0	9.0-13.0
10. Superior forefinger: As with forefinger grasp, but hand does not contact table; block is lifted deftly after grasp	13.0	13.0+

From *Genetic Psychology Monographs* 10:107, 1931. Reprinted with permission of the Helen Dwight Reid Educational Foundation. Published by Heldref Publishers, 4000 Albemarle St. NW, Washington, D.C. 20016. Copyright © 1931.

Observing Grasping Development

Age of the infant observed _____ months

Gender of infant _____ Time of day observed _____

Object placed in front of infant	Type of grip used on first offering	Type of grip used on second offering

From *Learning Activities for Life Span Motor Development Third Edition* by Kathleen Haywood and Nancy Getchell, 2001, Champaign, IL: Human Kinetics.

ACTIVITY 9.2

Assessing the Developmental Levels of Catchers

Purpose: To assess catching development in children and to observe the influence of varying ball size on the developmental level of catching.

Catching development typically lags behind that of the ballistic skills because catchers must anticipate where the ball or object can be intercepted and must move the hands, or even the entire body, to that position. It is a complex perceptual-motor task!

The goal of catching is to retain possession of the object caught. It is better to catch an object in the hands than to trap it against the body. The hands can better "give" to absorb force in order to retain the object. In games in which the object is to follow up a catch with another action, such as throwing, an object caught in the hands can be manipulated without delay. Young children, though, tend to trap the ball. Observations of catching focus on whether the ball is trapped or caught in the hands (see table 9.2 on p. 132 and the observation plan on p. 133). If the ball is trapped, we want to know whether the child is attempting to gather it by encircling it from the sides or scooping it from underneath. Our observations also focus on the hands and how they are positioned. Ideally, the palms face inward—fingers up for high balls, down for low balls—and adjust to the location where the ball will be intercepted. We also watch body movement to see whether the catcher adjusts to intercept the ball, and whether the movement comes before or after the catcher can determine the ball's flight.

The assessment of catching depends far more on environmental and task constraints than does assessment of locomotor and ballistic skills. For example, the size of the ball is critical. Even adults may resort to trapping a ball against the body if it is very large in relation to the hands. The direction of the oncoming ball can vary widely. The ball may be thrown directly to the catcher, a step away, or quite some distance away. Finally, the trajectory of the ball can vary, with high trajectories typically being more difficult for young or inexperienced catchers than flat trajectories. To compare individuals or to compare a single person's performance from time to time, we must be sure to note the environmental and task constraints established for the assessment and make sure they are consistent from catch to catch. For example, we might note that a Nerf ball 4 in. (10 cm) in diameter is thrown with a slight arc to 2 yd (2 m) either side of the catcher from a distance of 6.5 yd (6 m). In this observation, we will assess a catcher's developmental level with one set of conditions and then vary the size and weight of the ball to see how those changes affect performance.

Instructions

1. In this activity you will categorize catchers for their development levels of catching. Use the Developmental Sequence for Two-Handed Catching (table 9.2 on p. 132) and the observation plan on page 133 to guide your decisions on the catcher's arm, hand, and body action. First, categorize the catcher shown in the sequential still photos of figure 9.1. Next, on your CD-ROM, select the folder labeled Chapter 9 and then the folder labeled Catching. Work through the two examples in Set A. The program will prompt you to watch for the critical elements, just as in the observation plan. After completing Set A, categorize the examples in Set B. Label a column on record sheet 9.2 (p. 134) for each video example. You will have to follow the observation plan yourself this time. As you arrive at a

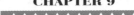

developmental level for each component, check that level in the appropriate column on record sheet 9.2.

2. After categorizing the photos and videos, arrange to categorize a child directly. It is ideal to do this assessment in pairs so that both you and your partner can toss the balls to be caught and can categorize the catcher. By warming up with the child, determine the distance from which you will toss, the trajectory you will use, and the locations around the catcher's starting position you will throw to (left, right, forward, back, and how far). Bring a variety of balls to the assessment, at least four in number. Balls should vary in size and weight from small (baseball sized) to large (playground/basketball sized). If the skill of your catcher is low, though, avoid using balls that would hurt the child if missed!

3. Toss approximately five times with each type of ball and categorize the catcher for each of the ball types. If a catcher performs at different levels on throws using the same ball, assign the level you observe most often (the modal level).

Questions

1. From the photos or videos, did you find catchers who were at different developmental levels in different body components? If so, describe. Did an older child or adult perform at a lower level than someone younger? If so, describe.

2. From your live observations, did your catcher perform at different levels on the five throws with a particular ball, or was your catcher consistent? If the catcher varied, did this seem to be a function of the throw itself (its trajectory and direction)? Explain.

3. What environmental constraints relating to the direction, distance, and trajectory of the ball flight produced the most difficult catching conditions for your performer?

4. Did changing the ball change the catcher's "developmental" level? How? Was the catcher less accurate in catching some balls compared to others? Why?

5. After your experience in this observation, what guidelines would you propose for those wishing to assess the developmental level of catching? Justify your suggestions.

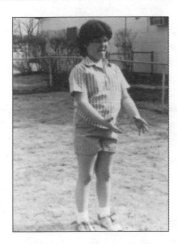 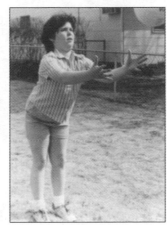 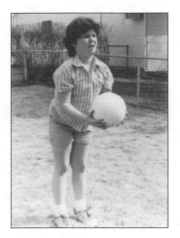

FIGURE 9.1 C.H., age 8.9 years, catching.

TABLE 9.2

Developmental Sequence for Two-Handed Catching

Arm action component

Step 1	Little response. Arms extend forward, but there is little movement to adapt to ball flight; ball is usually trapped against chest.
Step 2	Hugging. Arms are extended sideways to encircle the ball (hugging); ball is trapped against chest.
Step 3	Scooping. Arms are extended forward again but move under object (scoop); ball is trapped against chest.
Step 4	Arms "give." Arms extend to meet object with the hands; arms and body "give"; ball is caught in hands.

Hand action component

Step 1	Palms up. The palms of the hands face up. (Rolling balls elicit a palms-down, trapping action.)
Step 2	Palms in. The palms of the hands face each other.
Step 3	Palms adjusted. The palms of the hands are adjusted to the flight and size of the oncoming object. Thumbs or little fingers are placed close together, depending on the height of the flight path.

Body action component

Step 1	No adjustment. No adjustment of the body occurs in response to the ball's flight path.
Step 2	Awkward adjustment. The arms and trunk begin to move in relation to the ball's flight path but the head remains erect, creating an awkward movement to the ball. The catcher seems to be fighting to remain balanced.
Step 3	Proper adjustment. The feet, trunk, and arms all move to adjust to the path of the oncoming ball.

The arm action component is reprinted, by permission, from K.M. Haywood and N. Getchell., 2001, *Life span motor development*, 3rd ed. (Champaign, IL: Human Kinetics), 181, which is adapted from J.L. Haubenstricker, C.F. Branta, and V.D. Seefeldt, 1983, "Standards of Performance for Throwing and Catching." Paper presented at the annual conference of the North American Society for Psychology of Sport and Physical Activity, Asilomar, CA. Based on V. Seefeldt, S. Reuschlen, and P. Vogel, 1972, "Sequencing Motor Skills Within the Physical Education Curriculum." Paper presented at the annual conference of the American Association for Health, Physical Education and Recreation, Houston, TX. The hand and body action components are reprinted, by permission, from H.S. Strohmeyer, K. Williams, and D. Schaub-George, 1991, "Developmental sequences for catching a small ball: A prelongitudinal screening," *Research Quarterly for Exercise and Sport* 62: 259, 262.

OBSERVATION PLAN FOR CATCHING

ARM ACTION

Do the arms move to adapt to ball arrival?

- **No** → STEP 1 Little response
- **Yes** → Is the ball trapped against the chest or caught in the hands?
  - **Trapped** → STEP 2 or 3 Are the arms extended sideways to encircle ball or forward to scoop ball?
    - **Sideways** → STEP 2 Hugging
    - **Forward** → STEP 3 Scooping
  - **In hands** → STEP 4 Arms give

HAND ACTION

Do the palms face inward?

- **No** → STEP 1 Palms up/down
- **Yes** → Do the hands adjust to flight and size of ball (fingers pointed up for high level, down for low level)?
  - **No** → STEP 2 Palms inward
  - **Yes** → STEP 3 Hands adjustable

BODY ACTION

Does body move to adjust to flight of the ball?

- **No** → STEP 1 No adjustment
- **Yes** → Is body adjustment delayed to make an accurate movement?
  - **No** → STEP 2 Premature adjustment
  - **No** → STEP 3 Delayed adjustment

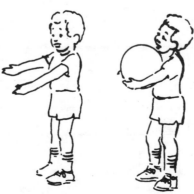

Arms, Step 3
Hands, Step 1
Body, Step 1

Assessing the Developmental Level of Catching

Observation Checklist: Catching

Observation number	1	2	3	4	5	6	7
Catcher's name, photo, or video number							
Catcher's age, if known							
Date							
Observation type*							
Component							
Arm action							
Step 1 Little response							
Step 2 Hugging							
Step 3 Scooping							
Step 4 Arms "give"							
Hand action							
Step 1 Palms up/down							
Step 2 Palms inward							
Step 3 Hands adjustable							
Body action							
Step 1 No adjustment							
Step 2 Premature adjustment							
Step 3 Delayed adjustment							
Summary profile							
Arm							
Hand							
Body							

*Codes for observation type: D = direct; P = photographs; F = film; V = video; S = slow motion.

From *Learning Activities for Life Span Motor Development Third Edition* by Kathleen Haywood and Nancy Getchell, 2001, Champaign, IL: Human Kinetics.

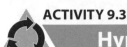

ACTIVITY 9.3

Hypothesizing Developmental Sequences

Purpose: To gain experience in hypothesizing a developmental sequence and to design an observation plan and checklist based on that hypothesized sequence.

In these last three chapters (chapters 7, 8, and 9), you have refined your observation techniques for many fundamental motor skills. You were provided with (1) developmental sequences that included detailed descriptions of each developmental level and (2) observation plans to guide your decisions. Developmental sequences, though, have not been validated—and sometimes not even hypothesized—for all the fundamental motor skills. What could you do in this case? It is possible to hypothesize a developmental sequence based on observations over an age range of performers. From a hypothesized sequence you can derive an observation plan and checklist. The sequence might not be as refined as one based on longitudinal research, but it might suit your purpose perfectly well.

In this activity you will have an opportunity to hypothesize a developmental sequence, an observation plan, and a checklist for kicking or some other skill for which there is no established developmental sequence. You will use your hypothesized assessment materials to see how well they work!

Instructions

1. Determine the skill for which you will hypothesize a sequence. Videos of kicking are provided on the CD-ROM, but your instructor may give you materials for some other skill or ask you to do an observation. If you decide to hypothesize a sequence for kicking, open your CD-ROM; open the folder labeled Chapter 9 and then the folder labeled Kicking. Watch each video several times as a background for hypothesizing a developmental sequence. If you know little about the skill for which you are hypothesizing a sequence or have not watched many learners perform the skill, research your skill before you hypothesize a developmental sequence.

2. Your first step is to decide which body components will have developmental sequences and whether separate components are needed for any phases of the skill (such as the windup in throwing or the ball-release phase in punting). Record your decisions on record sheet 9.3 (p. 137).

3. Your second step is to determine the developmental levels for each of the components. Give each level a number and title, and then describe the movement characteristic of that level on record sheet 9.3. Of course, you want to make the movement that is characteristic of the youngest performers "Step 1," the movement they would next achieve if you watched them develop over time "Step 2," and so on. Your last step should be the movement characteristic of the most developmentally advanced performers. There is no predetermined number of levels within each component, but obviously if you had more than three to five levels, your tool would be harder to use and more time consuming for those conducting an assessment.

4. On the basis of your developmental sequences for each component, design an observation plan on record sheet 9.4 (p. 138). Plan one component at a time. Try to design your observation plan so that one question is asked at a time, one decision is made at a time, and there are only two alternatives. Designate the angle from

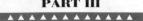
which the movement should be watched. You can include some stick-figure sketches in your plan to illustrate the movement that the decision focuses on.

5. On record sheet 9.5 (p. 139), create a checklist by entering the component, number, and titles of the sequential steps you identified.

6. Try out your observation plan and developmental sequence on three of the video clips. If your sequence or observation plan needs to be revised based on your categorizations of the performers in the video clips, make those revisions now.

7. Watch three to four performers of varying ages directly and categorize them according to your revised sequence and observation plan.

Questions

1. Were your initial sequence and observation plan workable for the performers on the video clips? What worked well? What problems did you encounter? What changes did you make in your sequence or observation plan?

2. Were your revised sequence and observation plan workable for direct observation of performers? What worked well? What problems did you encounter? On the basis of the direct observation, would you make any further revisions? If so, what changes are needed?

Hypothesizing Developmental Sequences

Developmental steps for the skill of _____

Body component _____

Step number	Title	Description

Body component _____

Step number	Title	Description

Body component _____

Step number	Title	Description

From *Learning Activities for Life Span Motor Development Third Edition* by Kathleen Haywood and Nancy Getchell, 2001, Champaign, IL: Human Kinetics.

Observation Plan for _____

Component _____

Component _____

Component _____

From *Learning Activities for Life Span Motor Development Third Edition* by Kathleen Haywood and Nancy Getchell, 2001, Champaign, IL: Human Kinetics.

Hypothesizing Developmental Sequences

Observation Checklist: _____

Observation number	1	2	3	4	5	6	7
Catcher's name, photo, or video number							
Catcher's age, if known							
Date							
Observation type*							
Component							
Step							
Step							
Step							
Step							
Step							
Step							
Step							
Step							
Step							
Step							
Step							
Step							
Step							
Step							
Step							

*Codes for observation type: D = direct; P = photographs; F = film; V = video; S = slow motion.

(continued)

From *Learning Activities for Life Span Motor Development Third Edition* by Kathleen Haywood and Nancy Getchell, 2001, Champaign, IL: Human Kinetics.

RECORD SHEET 9.5 *(continued)*

Observation number	1	2	3	4	5	6	7
Summary profile							

*Codes for observation type: D = direct; P = photographs; F = film; V = video; S = slow motion.

From *Learning Activities for Life Span Motor Development Third Edition* by Kathleen Haywood and Nancy Getchell, 2001, Champaign, IL: Human Kinetics.

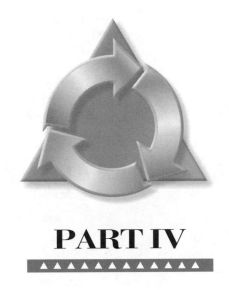

PART IV

Impact of Perceptual-Motor Development

CHAPTER 10

Sensory System Development

No matter which worldview we adopt, it is clear that individuals need information about the environment in order to move in that environment. Typically we distinguish sensation and perception. Sensation is the neural activity triggered by some stimulus that activates a sensory receptor and results in sensory nerve impulses' traveling the sensory nerve pathways to the brain. Perception is a multistage process that takes place in the brain and includes the selection, processing, organization, and integration of information received from the senses. Naturally, the perceptual process benefits from complete and accurate sensory information.

Developmentalists are interested in the development of the sensory systems during the growth period and changes in the sensory systems with aging. Is an individual getting the maximum information about the environment through the sensory systems? Or, must an individual compensate for a lack of information? If so, how is it that an individual compensates? In this chapter, you will have an opportunity to experience firsthand how you must adapt your behavior when sensory information is limited.

ACTIVITY 10.1

Moving in the Environment With Limited Sensation

Purpose: To experience moving and acting in the environment when information to one or more of the senses is limited.

Of all the sensory systems, vision, audition, and kinesthesis are the systems most involved in movement in and through the environment. You are probably familiar with

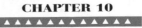

stories of individuals with sensory impairments who nevertheless are able to participate in sport and recreational activities. For example, there are individuals with blindness who snow ski, individuals who are deaf but who play professional football, and so on.

It might be hard for individuals with normal sensory system function to appreciate how people with sensory impairments must compensate in order to perform such feats. In this activity, you will have at least a limited opportunity to experience what it is like to move in the environment without all of the sensory information you are used to having!

Equipment List

Old sunglasses or eyeglass frames with one side covered over

Blindfold

Tennis ball

Basketball or playground ball

Earplugs/ear protectors

Whistle

Instructions

1. Work with a partner for these activities, so that one person can experience limited sensation while the other person guides and directs the activities. If time permits, reverse roles after each activity. Record your observations on record sheet 10.1 (p. 145).

2. First, you will participate in some activities with limited or no vision. Obtain an old pair of sunglasses without corrective lenses or old eyeglass frames, and cover one side such that you can see with only one eye. Using a tennis ball, play catch with your partner. Immediately afterward, note your impressions of participating under these conditions.

3. Obtain a blindfold. Position yourself in a hallway, place the blindfold over your eyes, and attempt to walk the length of the hallway with your partner watching to keep you safe. Using a basketball or playground ball, dribble the ball as you stand in position. After a while, attempt to walk the hallway as you dribble. Again, record your impressions.

4. Obtain a set of earplugs or the protectors worn by workers in noisy environments. Stand at one end of a long hallway, facing the end wall. Have your partner stand about 11 yd (10 m) behind you. Your partner should tell you to raise your hand if you can hear him or her. The partner should speak in a normal tone of voice and gradually increase the distance. Your partner should estimate the distance at which you could no longer hear the instruction. Repeat this activity outdoors with a whistle.

5. Still wearing your earplugs or protectors, sit in the back row of your classroom. Have your partner stand at the front and talk, sometimes turning to face a blackboard or the front wall. Take notes on what you understand of your partner's "speech."

6. Still wearing your earplugs or protectors, go to the hallway in your classroom building and place the blindfold over your eyes. Allow your partner to guide you through the building. Afterward, record your impressions of walking under these conditions.

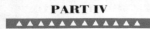
Questions

1. Covering one eye affects depth perception since we typically base our perceptions of depth on information from the two eyes. We can get clues about depth, though, from just one eye. How well did you catch with the vision from just one eye? Was the task more difficult than it would have been if you had had normal vision? Did you adopt any strategies for aiding your catching ability with just one eye? What sport, recreational, and everyday living activities would be affected if you had vision in only one eye?

2. How difficult was it to walk without vision? To dribble a ball standing still? To dribble a ball and walk? Did you improve with practice? How did you compensate for not being able to see?

3. At what distances could you no longer hear a speaking voice and a whistle when wearing earplugs? What sport, recreational, and everyday living activities would be affected by having limited hearing? How could someone participate in these activities; that is, what compensatory strategies could they use?

4. Could you pass a test on your partner's "speech" with limited hearing? How would the situation change in the various other classrooms and environments in which you have classes? Was it easy to "read lips" when you could not hear? What means are available today to allow those with limited hearing to compensate for this sensory loss?

5. Recount your impressions of walking without vision and only limited hearing. What feelings did you have?

Moving in the Environment With Limited Sensation

Catching with the use of one eye:

Walking blindfolded:

Hearing distance, spoken voice:

Hearing distance, whistle:

Taking notes with limited hearing:

Walking with no vision and limited hearing:

From *Learning Activities for Life Span Motor Development Third Edition* by Kathleen Haywood and Nancy Getchell, 2001, Champaign, IL: Human Kinetics.

CHAPTER 11

Perceptual-Motor Development

Have you ever heard different eyewitnesses give accounts of an automobile accident? Typically, each account is different—there will be some points that eyewitnesses agree on and other events that were noticed or are recalled by just one of the eyewitnesses. The varying accounts illustrate the difference between sensation and perception. Although all the individuals might have had the same sensations impinge on their sensory systems, they perceive those sensations somewhat differently. When individuals attach meaning to sensations, it quickly becomes clear that different individuals can interpret sensory stimuli in different ways.

If you consider the perception-action viewpoint, this should not be surprising. J.J. Gibson (1966, 1979) proposed that we actually perceive *affordances;* that is, we perceive the function that environmental objects, places, and events have for us. What those items afford can vary from individual to individual, based perhaps on the relative size of the individual and the items, an individual's goals, and so on. For example, let's say that an individual with a slight build sees a heavy sledgehammer lying on a table. We hand the person a nail and ask her to nail it into a piece of wood. She asks us for a hammer in order to undertake the task! She did not perceive that the heavy sledgehammer afforded her hammering. In contrast, a big, strong individual would merely pick up the sledgehammer to begin. So, individual and environment are so interactive as to be inseparable in determining functionality.

We know that the perceptual systems develop early in life. In many ways, it is not so difficult to isolate "perception" from the environment and to study the range of objects, sounds, events, and the like that can be perceived by an individual. If we do this we are using what is called a "reductionist" approach, looking at separate pieces to understand the whole. Much of what we know about perception and perceptual development was obtained through application of this approach. To perception-action developmentalists, the approach is artificial because they see the perceiving individual and the environment as an inseparable, integrated system. Yet developmentalists have not found very many ways to study perception and action as an ecosystem. Keep this in mind as you observe the development of perceptual-motor skills.

ACTIVITY 11.1

Testing Perceptual-Motor Development

Purpose: To become familiar with perceptual-motor test methods and to observe a child's performance on perceptual-motor tasks.

At times during the 20th century, developmentalists advocated screening children for perceptual-motor deficiencies in the belief that remediating such deficiencies would improve perceptual-cognitive skills. For example, they suggested that children without laterality (an ability to distinguish two sides of the body) and directionality (an ability to project that distinction into space) would also tend to reverse letters, such as **b** for **d**. Activities that improved this sense of "sides" would help children overcome this learning disability, so they thought. They promoted participation in early movement skill programs for this purpose.

Although research has failed to prove that such is the case, many of the screening tools these developmentalists designed remain useful in identifying children with perceptual-motor deficiencies. Teachers can use this information to plan perceptual-motor activities and lessons for children. These movement skill programs help children become more proficient movers. The published perceptual-motor surveys vary in content, often reflecting the author's emphasis. That is, one survey might have many items testing visual perception, another might emphasize sensory integration, and so on.

In this observation you will use a survey designed to familiarize you with some common ways to test visual, kinesthetic, and auditory perception. The survey does not have established reliability or validity, but it will show you how perceptual-motor development is tested.

Equipment List

Pencil

Low balance beam (or 8 ft [2.4 m] 2 × 4)

Three blocks of the same size but different colors

Small jingle bell

Life Span Motor Development text

Instructions

1. Give the test items on the survey as listed on record sheet 11.1 (pp. 149-150) to a child between 4 and 6 years of age. Your instructor may arrange for you to visit a school or program, or you will be asked to locate a young child on your own.

2. Obtain the child's birth date, and calculate a decimal age by adding to his/her age in years the number of months since his/her last birthday divided by 12 months. For example, if it is 6 months since a child's 5th birthday, the child is 5.5 years of age. Ask the child to write his or her name so you can determine the dominant hand. Record this information on record sheet 11.1.

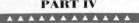
3. Conduct the tests for visual, kinesthetic, and auditory perception according to the instructions given at the beginning of each test item. Before conducting each test, briefly explain it to the child. Record your results in the spaces provided.

Questions

1. Which aspects of perceptual-motor development seemed to be well developed in the child with whom you worked? Which perceptual-motor discriminations must yet be refined? Cite results to support your answer.

2. Did vision, kinesthesis, and audition seem to be equally developed? What do you base your answer on?

3. According to the age ranges for perceptual development provided in your text or background reading, do your results seem appropriate for the age of the child you observed? Why or why not?

4. Were any test items difficult to explain to the child or to score? Would you change any of the test items? If so, how? If not, why?

Testing Perceptual-Motor Development

Child writes first name _____

Sex _____ Birth date _____ Decimal age _____ Dominant hand: R   L

I. Visual Perception: Size Constancy and Spatial Orientation

Arrange three blocks on a long table, about 3 ft (0.9 m) from the child, so that they are spread out away from the child, about 6 in. (15 cm) apart. After the first four questions, bring the blocks directly in front of the child. Ask questions or give instructions as follows, and record whether or not the response was correct.

Question/direction	Correct	Incorrect
1. What color is this? (Do each block.)		
2. Which block is closest to you?		
3. Which block is the farthest away?		
4. Are the blocks the same size?		
5. Place the blocks so that the blue block is higher than the yellow block.		
6. Place the blue block so that it is lower than the yellow block but higher than the red block.		

Number correct _____/6

II. Visual Perception: Whole and Parts

Using figure 11.4 in *Life Span Motor Development,* point to one of the pictures in the figure. Ask the child what the picture shows. Record whether the child describes the parts (fruit, candy, etc.), the whole picture (a face), or both (a scooter made out of candy). Point to a second picture, and repeat the question. Record the category of response.

1. _____ Parts _____ Whole _____ Both

2. _____ Parts _____ Whole _____ Both

III. Kinesthetic perception: Identification of Body Parts

Give the instructions listed, and record whether the child touches the correct or incorrect body part.

Direction	Correct	Incorrect
1. Touch your nose.		
2. Touch your hips.		
3. Touch your wrists.		

From *Learning Activities for Life Span Motor Development Third Edition* by Kathleen Haywood and Nancy Getchell, 2001, Champaign, IL: Human Kinetics.

(continued)

Direction	Correct	Incorrect
4. Touch your knees.		
5. Touch your heels.		
6. Touch your ears.		
7. Touch your shoulders.		

Number correct _____/7

IV. Kinesthetic Perception: Left/Right Discrimination

Give the instructions listed and record whether the response is correct or incorrect.

Direction	Correct	Incorrect
1. Touch your right ear.		
2. Touch your left knee.		
3. Pick up this pencil with your left hand.		
4. Is the pencil on your right or left? (Place the pencil on the right.)		
5. Touch your left hip with your right hand.		

Number correct _____/5

V. Kinesthetic Perception: Balance

Position the child at one end of a low balance beam, with both feet on the beam. Ask the child to walk along the beam to the other end without falling off. Record the number of steps the child takes before stepping off the beam and whether the beam walk was completed.

Number of steps _____ Walk completed? _____ Yes _____ No

VI. Auditory Perception: Location

Holding a small jingle bell, face the child and place both hands behind your back. Place the bell in one hand, and form a fist with each hand to conceal the bell's location. Bring your hands to the front, keep them about 8 in. apart, and shake them to make the bell jingle. Ask the child to point to the hand holding the bell. Repeat four more times, randomly placing the bell in either hand.

	Correct	Incorrect
1.		
2.		
3.		
4.		
5.		

Number correct _____/5

From *Learning Activities for Life Span Motor Development Third Edition* by Kathleen Haywood and Nancy Getchell, 2001, Champaign, IL: Human Kinetics.

ACTIVITY 11.2

Development of Intermodal Perception

Purpose: To observe intermodal perception in a child by asking the child to match objects perceived through vision and kinesthesis.

In applying the reductionist approach to study perception, it is easy to forget that it is typically an event that we perceive. A book falling to the floor can be seen and heard; a mosquito biting can be seen and felt! Perceptions in the various systems are obviously brought together, such that we know a sight, sound, or feel is the same event even though it is perceived in multiple modalities. This is termed intermodal perception or sensory integration.

The information-processing and perception–action perspectives have different ways of considering intermodal perception. The information-processing perspective recognizes that the stimulus to each system is a different form of energy—light waves, sound waves, temperature, and so on. So each sensory system registers a unique sensation and perception. The task of a developing infant is to learn how to integrate the separate systems—to learn how those unique sensations are related to one another.

The perception–action perspective sees the sensory-perceptual systems as united in bringing information about events to the individual, just through different modalities. The perceptual systems extract patterns. The task of a developing infant is to learn about events in the world.

Regardless of the perspective we prefer to take, much of the research on intermodal perception has been conducted from the information-processing perspective. In this observation we will use a method consistent with this perspective to learn more about visual-kinesthetic intermodal perception.

Equipment List

Six small objects—for example, a block, a small ball, a toy car. Objects should be relatively simple in shape.

Instructions

1. Work with a child approximately 5 years of age. Have the child sit at a table and push his or her chair forward such that the hands, if held in the lap, are not visible to the child.

2. Place three of the objects on the table and let the child see but not touch them. After a few minutes, take these three away and mix them with the three objects the child has not seen.

3. One by one and in random order, hand the child the objects under the table so he or she can feel and manipulate the object. Ask the child if the object is one of those previously seen on the table. Record the answers on record sheet 11.2 (p. 153). Ask the child how he or she decided those were the right objects.

4. Repeat this exercise but with the order reversed. Select three of the objects and present them one by one under the table so that the child can spend about a minute manipulating each one. Place all six on the top of the table and ask the child to point to the three he or she has manipulated sight unseen.

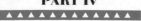

Questions

1. Considering the accuracy of the child in identifying the objects, was the child more accurate when the objects were presented first visually or first kinesthetically, or was the child equally accurate with either vision or kinesthesis first?

2. Were there some objects that were more difficult for the child to identify than others? If so, why do you think this was the case? If not, why not?

3. Research studies have shown that presenting objects first visually makes for an easier intermodal perception task than presenting objects first kinesthetically. To arrive at this conclusion, researchers would observe many children, with half seeing the objects first and the other half feeling the objects first. In our observation, the child had an opportunity to become familiar with the objects in the visual-kinesthetic task before attempting the kinesthetic-visual task. Do you think this was a factor in the outcome? Why or why not?

4. From the answers your child gave to your question about how he/she decided on the objects, what can you say about the information the child used in the decision? For example, did the child report using sharp edges or smooth surfaces to make the decision?

5. On the basis of the learning activity, can you think of everyday situations in which it benefits teachers or parents to know the course of intermodal perception?

The Development of Intermodal Perception

Child's decimal age _____ Child's sex _____

I. V-K (Visual first, Kinesthetic second) Task

The three objects presented visually: _____

The three objects the child identified kinesthetically: _____

Strategies reported by the child:

II. K-V Task

The three objects presented kinesthetically: _____

The three objects the child identified visually: _____

Strategies reported by the child:

From *Learning Activities for Life Span Motor Development Third Edition* by Kathleen Haywood and Nancy Getchell, 2001, Champaign, IL: Human Kinetics.

CHAPTER 12

Perception and Action in Development

In recent years the information-processing perspective and the systems perspective have dominated research in motor development. The systems perspective has two branches: the dynamic systems branch, which addresses how movements are organized and controlled, and the ecological, or perception–action, branch, which addresses how movement and perception interrelate.

The information-processing perspective tends to view movement as a response to the perceptual information taken in by the sensory-perceptual systems and processed by the cognitive systems. Movement and perception, then, are viewed as distinct and separate. The ecological, or perception–action, perspective, on the other hand, sees perception and movement, or action, as so interrelated as to be indistinguishable. The movements that environmental places, objects, and events afford an individual actually define their function. A chair has the function of "sitting on" for us only if the seat is about 20 in. (50 cm) off the ground. It does not have the function of sitting on if the seat is 60 in. (150 cm) off the ground! So the "perception" of an object or surface and the movements related to it are inseparable.

For those who prefer the ecological, or perception–action, perspective, several movement situations are exemplars for the interrelationship of perception and action. First, those who hold this perspective point to the apparent need for infants to undertake self-produced locomotion to develop a sense of spatial relationships. Second, they stress the ways movement changes as environmental objects and surfaces are scaled to body size. Finally, they discuss postural control and balance as an ecosystem. Here, we first will observe balance and the interrelationship of perception and movement.

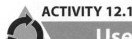

ACTIVITY 12.1

Use of Light Touch in Maintaining Balance

Purpose: To observe the interaction of perception and movement in maintaining balance.

Maintaining a desired posture and our overall balance seems simple to many of us. Once past infancy, we take for granted the thousands of small adjustments our bodies make to maintain posture and balance. We do not give this a second thought unless we are in a precarious balance situation, such as walking on ice or moving through a "haunted" house that presents conflicting information to our senses. Only in older adulthood, in the presence of disease or declining skeletal and muscle strength, does balance once again become an issue for activities of daily living.

If we think more carefully about maintaining posture and balance, we realize that this is indeed a complex process. To maintain posture and balance, we must continually change our motor response patterns according to the perceptual information that specifies the environment and our body's orientation in it. The perceptual information comes from several perceptual systems and almost countless sensory receptors! Vision tells us how our body is positioned in the environment. Kinesthesis tells us how our limbs and body parts are positioned relative to each other and about our head position and movement. Even the auditory system can contribute information about balance. So, there is a constant interaction of perceptual information and action to maintain our posture and balance.

Jeka has shown that adults can use information from light touches of the hand on surrounding surfaces to monitor and minimize body sway (Jeka, 1998; Jeka & Lackner, 1994, 1995). These are forces much smaller than one would use for support. They are just large enough to enhance perception. That is, they are not a reaction to a threat to balance but rather are information used in an interactive way to control posture. Barela, Jeka, and Clark (1999) observed that infants can use touch information after they have acquired some walking experience. In this observation we will see whether light-touch information helps toddlers maintain their balance.

Equipment List

A 2 × 4 at least 2 ft (61 cm) long

A table approximately 18 to 21 in. (46-53 cm) high

A table 27 to 30 in. (69-76 cm) high

A stopwatch

Instructions

1. Locate two children between the ages of 3 and 5 years and two of your classmates. You can observe the participants one at a time.

2. Place the 2 × 4 on the floor, 4 in. side down.

3. First ask each of your participants to stand toe-to-heel on the 2 × 4 and to maintain his/her balance for as long as possible. Time them from their start until they step off the board. Record the time on record sheet 12.1 (p. 157). Repeat twice for a total of three times.

4. Then, place the appropriate table (shorter for the children, higher for the adults) next to the board. Ask your participants to now stand on the board as before, but

tell them that they may place the fingertips of their nearest hand on the table. Stress that they are not to push down on the table, but just touch it lightly (see figure 12.1). Time them again, from start either to step-off or until you see them push on the table for support. Record the time on record sheet 12.1. Repeat twice for a total of three times.

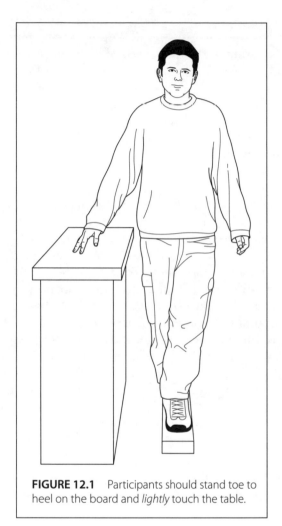

FIGURE 12.1   Participants should stand toe to heel on the board and *lightly* touch the table.

Questions

1. Looking at the average times and on the whole, do you find that your participants balanced longer with or without light touch? Were there individuals who were exceptions to the group results?

2. Did either group, the children or the adults, benefit more than the other group from light touch—that is, did one group do *much* better in the touch condition? On what do you base your answer?

3. Why do you think light-touch information would help someone balance longer? Can you think of circumstances in everyday life in which people seek light-touch information to maintain balance? Did you observe any indications that individuals were using light touch to maintain their balance rather than reacting to losing balance? What were these indications?

Use of Light Touch in Maintaining Balance

Participant	Condition	Trial 1	Trial 2	Trial 3	Average
Child #1	No touch				
	Light touch				
Child #2	No touch				
	Light touch				
Adult #1	No touch				
	Light touch				
Adult #2	No touch				
	Light touch				

	No-touch averages		Light-touch averages
Child #1	_____	vs.	_____
Child #2	_____	vs.	_____
Adult #1	_____	vs.	_____
Adult #2	_____	vs.	_____

From *Learning Activities for Life Span Motor Development Third Edition* by Kathleen Haywood and Nancy Getchell, 2001, Champaign, IL: Human Kinetics.

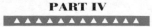

ACTIVITY 12.2

Body Scaling for Promoting Safety

Purpose: To identify ways in which engineers, manufacturers, and developmentalists use body scaling to increase safety.

Earlier, in our introduction, we acknowledged that developmentalists who adopt the ecological perspective stress the ways in which movement changes as environmental objects and surfaces are scaled to body size. For example, ecologists see stair climbing in infants as a question of scale—the height or rise of the stairs in relation to the size of the infant's body. Consider an infant who crawls up stairs or a toddler who uses a "mark time" pattern (placing the lead foot on a stair, then bringing the rear foot to the same stair instead of to the next higher or lower stair as adults do). Ecologists do not say that the infant or toddler has not "learned" to climb stairs correctly. Rather, they see this as a natural movement solution to the problem of ascending and descending stairs with step heights that are suited to (that is, scaled to) adult-sized bodies! If the child is presented with a set of stairs with short step heights, or when the child grows and the body is not so small compared to step heights, the stairs then afford the child the alternate stepping pattern that adults use. You can experiment with a similar situation yourself if you know where there is a spiral staircase. A spiral staircase necessarily varies the depth (width) of each step. The stepping surface must be narrow near the center and wide at the edge. Try going up and down these stairs to see where you can ascend or descend with a normal, alternating pattern; where it is almost more comfortable to take two stairs at a time; and where you revert to the mark time pattern used by infants.

It is tempting always to look at examples of body scaling in terms of adaptations that afford, or *permit*, a developing individual to do *more*. That is, can shortening a racket permit a child to strike a ball? Can we lower a basketball goal to permit a youth to use a jump shot? Can we make a bicycle smaller to permit riding by a small child? Yet many engineers, inventors, manufacturers, and safety specialists are equally concerned with determining how to scale spaces, surfaces, and objects to prevent an activity! In the following learning activity we will explore some situations in which this is the goal.

Instructions

1. Work either individually or with a small group of classmates as your instructor indicates. As your first step, think of at least three ways in which someone has adapted spaces to prevent a particular movement or action, and three ways in which someone has adapted surfaces to prevent a movement or action. Then, think of at least three objects that have been modified to prevent their use in an unsafe way. (Hints: Think about fences; think about surfaces near water or ice.) Record your reflections on record sheet 12.2 (p. 160).

2. Using a search engine on the World Wide Web, identify three organizations or government agencies that have determined or that promote guidelines for modifying spaces, surfaces, and objects to increase safety and reduce risk. That is, find three organizations concerned with risk management. Classify them as to whether their major concerns are spaces, surfaces, or objects. Enter the names of your organizations and their classifications on record sheet 12.2.

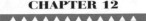
Questions

1. Consider the modified or adapted spaces, surfaces, and objects you initially identified. Describe how each is scaled to the size of an adult or child.

2. Did any of the organizations you located address the modifications you initially identified? If so, which ones and in what ways? If not, what organizations do you think might address your modifications?

3. Were you able to find detailed specifications for how spaces, surfaces, or objects should be constructed or arranged to prevent certain movements? For example, did any organization address the distances between vertical posts in constructing a deck railing or fence?

4. What was most often the type of movement someone was trying to prevent? For example, was it climbing, crawling through, falling?

5. Select an environment or situation in which a teacher or therapist works with students or clients. What places or objects in this environment are likely to be modified to promote safety and reduce risk as individuals go about their daily routines?

Reflections on Body Scaling for Promoting Safety

Category	Describe the modifications
Spaces	1. 2. 3.
Surfaces	1. 2. 3.
Objects	1. 2. 3.

Organization/agency	Web address	Modifies spaces, surfaces, or objects?

From *Learning Activities for Life Span Motor Development Third Edition* by Kathleen Haywood and Nancy Getchell, 2001, Champaign, IL: Human Kinetics.

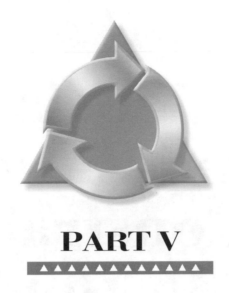

PART V

Impact of Functional Constraints

CHAPTER 13

Social and Cultural Constraints in Motor Development

Society and culture can have a profound effect on an individual's movement behaviors, particularly in the area of sport and physical activity (Clark, 1994). In fact, these factors act as environmental constraints. That is, sociocultural attitudes of groups of people act to either encourage or discourage certain motor behaviors. Why do we consider these to be environmental constraints? The reason is that they reflect a general attitude, or belief system, that is present in society at large or within certain subcultures. If these attitudes are pervasive enough (since they can be subtle yet powerful), they can modify someone's behavior. Just as temperature or ambient light can encompass a room, field, or community, so can attitudes, values, norms, or stereotypes.

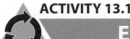

ACTIVITY 13.1

Examining Gender Role Stereotyping

Purpose: To examine the packaging of toys and television commercials for evidence of gender role stereotyping.

Most of us are so used to the advertising and marketing messages impinging on us daily that we neglect to question the assumptions underlying them. Recall from the discussion in chapter 13 of your textbook that toys are a facet of the socialization process. The manner in which toys are marketed to children both reflects societal attitudes and tends to maintain them. This is particularly true with regard to gender roles. Manufacturers find it advantageous to market their products with sex-typed strategies. This learning activity will prompt you to examine toy-marketing strategies and to decide whether these strategies socialize children into traditional gender roles.

Instructions

1. Visit a local toy store or the toy section in a department store. Evaluate 20 different children's toys and how they are packaged. On record sheet 13.1, enter each toy's name, its category (sedentary game, construction toy, etc.), the key word or phrase used by the manufacturer to market the toy (e.g., "just like Mom's"), whether boys or girls are pictured on the package, and the children's approximate ages.

2. Watch two children's programs on television. Choose a time slot popular for children's viewing rather than family viewing. Observe the commercials during and immediately following each program. Using record sheet 13.2 (p. 165), record the name of every toy advertised, the type, the key marketing phrase used, and whether boys or girls are pictured in the commercial.

Questions

1. Consider the category of toy in both the toy stores and the commercials. Do you find a tendency for girls to be shown with toys related to a domestic role or to mothering, whereas boys are shown with toys related to action careers? On what do you base your answer? If you find this tendency, do you believe it serves a useful purpose? If so, how do you believe this influences boys and girls to choose certain careers?

2. If you examined any sport-equipment toys, were boys or girls pictured? Cite examples. Did the type of sport make a difference? How?

3. Consider the category of toy again. Was there a tendency for either sex to be associated with games or toys for sedentary play? For active play? Cite examples. What implications might these tendencies have for the skill development and physical fitness of children?

4. What other differences did you observe in the way specific types of toys were marketed to subgroups (sex, age, cultural group, etc.) of children?

5. On the basis of your observations in this activity, do you believe that toys are a part of the socialization process, especially socialization into gender roles? On what findings do you base your answer?

Toy Store Visit

Name of toy	Toy category[a]	Key marketing phrase	Children pictured (age, sex)

[a]Examples: construction/building set, sedentary game, make-believe domestic role (e.g., kitchen set), make-believe action career (e.g., soldier), educational toy/computer, sport equipment.

From *Learning Activities for Life Span Motor Development Third Edition* by Kathleen Haywood and Nancy Getchell, 2001, Champaign, IL: Human Kinetics.

Television Commercials

Name of toy	Toy category[a]	Key marketing phrase	Sexes of children pictured

[a]Examples: construction/building set, sedentary game, make-believe domestic role (e.g., kitchen set), make-believe action career (e.g., soldier), educational toy/computer, sport equipment.

From *Learning Activities for Life Span Motor Development Third Edition* by Kathleen Haywood and Nancy Getchell, 2001, Champaign, IL: Human Kinetics.

ACTIVITY 13.2

Observing Sociocultural Constraints on the World Wide Web

Purpose: To use the Internet to explore sociocultural constraints in six different countries.

One of the benefits of the World Wide Web is that Americans, as well as people in other countries, have immediate access to information about many different societies and cultures. After a little Web browsing, it becomes clear that different societies and cultures promote different activities for their members. You will find diverse sports in which people participate, various ages at which certain activities are deemed appropriate, different roles for males and females, and so on. For this learning activity, you will use the Internet to explore several different countries, and then determine their specific sociocultural constraints.

Instructions

1. In this learning activity, you will discover what your motor development might have been like if you had grown up in a different society and culture. To do this, you will assume the role of a college-aged individual from each of the six continents. First, select a country from each of six different continents (Africa, Asia, Australia, Europe, North America, and South America). Choose a country other than the one in which you reside.

2. Next, visit *at least* two Web sites *from* each country as well as two Web sites *about* each country (for example, from an encyclopedia or travel guide). Remember to record these Web sites for future reference. Also, the more Web sites you visit, the more information you will have with which to work!

3. For each country, try to determine what sociocultural constraints exist. The following questions will help you guide your search, but do not feel limited to them!

   - What are some of the physical constraints from the environment that may affect motor development?

   - What are the types of games that are played in each country?

   - What types of sports are played? Focus on sports with which you are not familiar.

   - Are there any culturally specific values or rules that are apparent?

   - What types of clothing are acceptable and for whom?

   - What is the school system like?

4. Develop a biographical composite of yourself had you been born and raised in each of the countries you chose. Focus on sociocultural constraints. What would you be like? How would your life and motor development differ from country to country? Would there be similarities in physical activities, exercise, movements, and sports among the countries? Finally, how would your different, hypothetical motor development compare to your actual motor development?

CHAPTER 14

Psychosocial Constraints in Motor Development

People choose to engage in or avoid various types of motor behaviors for many reasons. Whether we realize it or not, our social surround can influence individual feelings about physical activities, especially over a period of time. Emotions such as self-esteem, motivation, and attributions of success or failure develop from an interaction between individual (functional) and environmental (sociocultural) constraints. Remember that a functional individual constraint is not a specific anatomical structure, but more like a psychological construct such as motivation, self-efficacy, or emotions. Often, socializing agents such as parents or peers play a strong role in developing these functional individual constraints. Therefore, here we will consider the interaction between sociocultural constraints and functional individual constraints.

As you explored in chapter 13, the social or cultural environment can act to encourage or discourage various movement behaviors. These environmental constraints may affect different individuals in unique ways, depending on how various constraints have interacted in the past. In the following learning activities, we will explore the interaction between social factors and functional constraints, such as self-esteem, perceived ability, motivation, and other personal attributes.

ACTIVITY 14.1

Identifying Causal Attributions in Sport Participants

Purpose: To identify the reasons individuals give for success or failure when participating in sport.

Self-esteem can influence behavior because people tend to act in ways that confirm their beliefs about themselves; that is, people tend to be *self-consistent*. Individuals with low perceived competency and low self-esteem surrounding their ability to perform movement skills tend to perform the skill with low competency. Those with higher self-esteem tend to perform with higher competency. Beliefs of competency may be determined by the reasons people give for their successes and failures, called causal attributions. These reasons differ for people with high and low self-esteem. According to Weiner (1986), these causal attributions fit into a three-dimensional framework, which establishes differences in attributional patterns between high and low achievers. The first of the three dimensions is locus of control, which can be internal (ability or amount of effort) or external (difficulty of the task, luck). Stability is the next dimension, which can be stable (ability) or unstable (officiating). The third dimension, controllability, relates to whether something is under the control of the individual or others (effort) or is not controllable (task difficulty, officiating) (see table 14.1). Individuals who have high self-esteem tend to attribute outcomes to factors that are internal, stable, and controllable (e.g. effort), whereas those with lower self-esteem attribute outcomes to factors that are external, unstable, and uncontrollable (luck).

TABLE 14.1

Dimension	High achiever	Low achiever
Locus of causality	Internal ("I played my best.")	External ("We were lucky.")
Stability	Stable ("I have a great shot.")	Unstable ("I didn't try my hardest.")
Controllability	Controllable ("We didn't work together as well as we could have.")	Uncontrollable ("The officials called everything for the other team.")

Instructions

For this activity, you will interview four individuals, two on a youth sport team and two on an intercollegiate team. You will attempt to determine where each individual lies on Weiner's three-dimensional attributional framework.

1. Pick a sport in which you are interested, one for which you have access to interviewees.

2. For your first two interviews, find a successful youth sport team in your sport. Find two players whom you can interview separately, one right after the other (so that the players do not converse about the interview).

3. Repeat this process for the second two interviews with intercollegiate players. Again, interview the two separately, one right after the other.

4. For your interviews, ask questions that will help you to understand the interviewees' causal attributions for success or failure. We have provided a list of general questions, but you should not feel limited by these questions; modify them according to the sport, or add any that are relevant. Record sheet 14.1 is the interview sheet.

5. When you are finished with your interviews, evaluate the answers to see where they fall in terms of the attribution dimensions. For example, if an athlete answers the question, "Why did your team win?" with the statement, "We got lucky; the other team was better," then the attribution is external, unstable, and uncontrollable. When asked about the relationship between a team's loss and personal play, a response of, "We all tried as hard as we could," represents attribution that is internal, stable, and controllable.

6. Answer the following discussion questions.

Questions

1. Where did each individual lie in terms of causal attributions? Remember to examine all three dimensions.

2. Compare and contrast the two athletes within each team. Did their attributions differ? Why?

3. Compare and contrast the athletes across the teams. Do you detect any developmental differences in attributions? Any similarities between the players? What might account for the similarities and differences?

4. Make inferences about each individual's self-esteem based on causal attributions. Compare and contrast self-esteem across teams. Do you detect any developmental differences?

Causal Attributions Interview

Name _____ Age _____ Amount of experience _____

Sport _____ Position(s) played _____

Team name _____ Record _____

1. Think about the last game that your team won. What were the primary reasons that your team won?

2. Think about your performance in that game. What was the relationship between your play and the team's win?

3. Think about the last game that your team lost. What were the primary reasons that your team lost?

4. Think about your performance in that game. What was the relationship between your play and the team's loss?

5. In both of these games, could anything have changed that would have altered the outcome of these games?

6. In both of these games, could changes in your performance have had any influence on the outcome of these games?

7. [Add your own sport- or individual-specific questions.]

From *Learning Activities for Life Span Motor Development Third Edition* by Kathleen Haywood and Nancy Getchell, 2001, Champaign, IL: Human Kinetics.

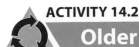

ACTIVITY 14.2

Older Adults' Persistence in Physical Activities

Purpose: To examine the psychosocial constraints that lead to older adults' participation and persistence in physical activities.

As we've discussed in the *Life Span Motor Development* text (chapter 14 and the chapters on physical fitness), participating in physical activities across the life span leads to improved physical and emotional well-being. Yet older adults tend to decrease their activity levels or even drop out of physical activities as a result of the interaction of several influential constraints. The aging process leads to changes in structural constraints (many of which can be reversed through physical activity), such as weight gain, muscle weakness, and joint pain. These structural changes can result in changes in functional constraints, such as fear, decreased motivation, and decreased self-esteem. In terms of sociocultural constraints, older adults in the United States have suffered in the past few decades from a cultural perception of frailty; this leads to fewer opportunities in physical activity and sport. All of these constraints interact to result in declining rates of physical activity in older adults.

Perhaps this picture of older adults and physical activity seems rather pessimistic. In fact, the perception of older adults as frail has been challenged frequently in the past several years. Consider the book of photographs titled *Growing Old Is Not for Sissies* by Etta Clark, which portrays older adult athletes; or think about the Senior Olympic movement, which has increased participation year after year. More and more seniors are becoming physically active. It will help us to encourage older adults to participate if we have a better understanding of why older adults do participate and persist in physical activities. We should understand how physical activity instructors modify constraints within activities so that seniors can participate fully. Further, we must learn what motivates senior participants to stick with physical activities. What better way to do this than to interview an older adult who participates in physical activities!

Instructions

1. Find a local group or program that provides physical activities to older adults. Often, the local YMCA or YWCA has programs specifically for seniors. Also, many universities have "lifelong learning" or similar activity programs in which many older adults participate.

2. Make sure you contact the instructor prior to your observation in order to get permission to watch the class. If at all possible, participate in the class; this will give you a greater understanding of the activities involved.

3. When you are not participating, position yourself so that you can observe the participants without making them feel self-conscious. Watch carefully, keeping in mind the various individual, environmental, and task constraints and how they all interact.

4. After the class, interview one or more of the participants. Spend at least 15 min talking to people about their motor development and physical fitness history. Ask them how long they've participated, why they participate, about fitness benefits, about injuries or conditions they might have, and the like. Try to get a good feel for the constraints encouraging or discouraging their behaviors.

5. Use your observations and your interviews to answer the following questions.

Questions

1. What are the activities in which the older adults participate?

2. What seem to be the most important individual constraints affecting these individuals?

3. Describe several ways that the instructor has modified the task or environmental constraints to accommodate the individual constraints of these older individuals. Be specific.

4. How are the older adults responding to the class? Do they seem to be participating fully? Do they appear to modify their motor behaviors because of particular task or environmental constraints?

5. What other modifications or activities could an instructor make in order to create a successful program for seniors? Consider the entire spectrum of constraints.

CHAPTER 15

Knowledge As a Functional Constraint in Motor Development

It is easy to overlook the role of knowledge in the performance of motor skills. In fact, knowledge is an individual, functional constraint. The knowledge a performer brings to a situation interacts with task and environmental constraints. An expert is likely to move differently than a novice, even when faced with identical environmental and task constraints. A performer with little knowledge of a sport game might be slow in moving or perform an incorrect movement for the goal of the task. A knowledgeable performer recognizes patterns quickly, makes fast decisions, and analyzes problems at an advanced level.

The amount of information a person possesses on a specific topic is called his/her *knowledge base*. The knowledge base contains declarative knowledge (i.e., factual information) and possibly procedural knowledge (i.e., information about how to do something) and strategic knowledge (i.e., general rules or strategies). Obviously, experts have more knowledge, or a larger knowledge base, than novices. Experts also structure their information differently than novices. They organize information in a methodical structure. This likely helps them access and use their information more efficiently than a novice would. The manner in which a person organizes information about a topic is called his/her knowledge structure.

Expertise is specific: having much knowledge of one topic makes a person an expert on that topic but does not guarantee that person is an expert on any other topic, even if it is related. So, in order to perform well in a sport or dance form, a performer must have both knowledge and physical skill. In these observations, you will interview performers of different ages to determine their knowledge structure in a particular sport.

ACTIVITY 15.1

The Knowledge Structure of a Youth Sport Participant

Purpose: To discover how much declarative knowledge a youth sport participant has about his or her sport.

Children typically are novices in any area, including sport and dance. They must build a knowledge base, beginning with declarative knowledge. They must learn the game rules, goals, and strategies necessary to perform in a sport or dance form. Then they can acquire procedural knowledge and learn to make appropriate decisions about which actions to perform. Strategic knowledge is probably the last to develop, since it requires experience in many types of tasks within a given activity. Research has demonstrated that over a short term, individual children can perform better not so much because their physical skills have improved rapidly, but because they have learned more about their sport (French & Thomas, 1987). So, increasing knowledge is a benefit to youth sport participants.

Some children do become experts on a particular topic, even at a young age. Youth sport experts can demonstrate more knowledge of a sport and generate more tactical concepts about that sport than adult novices! Remember, though, that experience in playing is important in developing a knowledge structure. A child who knows about a sport—perhaps quoting statistics and anecdotes about players—but who has not played the sport still does not possess the knowledge structure that would help her perform well.

In this observation you will interview a youth sport participant who has played for several years in order to determine his or her knowledge structure for that sport.

Instructions

1. Locate a youth sport participant, approximately 12 or 13 years old, who has been playing baseball, softball, basketball, or soccer for at least 4 or 5 years. You need approximately 20 to 30 min to interview your athlete. Tell the athlete that you would like to find how much he/she knows about the sport.

2. Your interview initially should focus on determining the athlete's declarative knowledge, factual information about the skills of the sport. Declarative knowledge is easier to verbalize than procedural or strategic knowledge. For this interview, we will not seek knowledge about the history of the sport, training or conditioning, or the psychosocial concepts related to the sport. When you have finished with questions about the skills of the sport, ask your youth sport participant about the strategies of the sport. That is, determine his or her strategic knowledge of the sport.

3. As you interview your athlete you should record his or her knowledge about the sport as a hierarchy. This hierarchy is started for you on record sheet 15.1 (p. 176). You might want to sketch the hierarchy on a separate sheet of paper, using a pencil, during the interview and then transpose it onto record sheet 15.1 at a later time. You also can audiotape the interview if that is acceptable to the athlete. It is acceptable for the athlete to see the hierarchy.

4. A basic interview format is suggested here, but you should be flexible with your interview questions. Some athletes will volunteer more information than others. You might need to ask some athletes more follow-up questions than others.

- What are the individual offensive skills in [add sport]? (You are looking for skills such as dribbling in soccer, jump shot in basketball, bunting in baseball/softball; as the athlete names the skills, put each in a box under "Offensive" under "Skills." See record sheet 15.1.)

- What are the individual defensive skills in [sport]? (You are looking for skills such as guarding in basketball, marking in soccer, catching fly balls in baseball/softball; as the athletes names the skills, put each in a box under "Defensive" under "Skills.")

- For each offensive and defensive skill, determine whether the athlete can break the skill into subskills by asking, "Do you know any 'parts' of [skill]?" (You are determining, for example, if a soccer player says passing is an offensive skill, whether he/she knows an instep pass, an outside-foot pass, and the like. If so, extend a line from the "Passing" box down, draw a horizontal line, then extend lines and draw boxes below them for instep pass, outside-foot pass, and so on. Always add as many boxes and lines as you need to record all the athlete knows.)

- If time permits, you also can ask whether the athlete knows any important points of technique for the subskills named. Examples are keeping the elbow in on a basketball jump shot, moving to get in front of a ground ball when catching in baseball/softball.

- What are the offensive strategies in [sport]? (You are looking for patterns of play, such as a "give and go" in soccer or basketball, or bunting so a base runner can move from first base to second base in baseball/softball. Record these as before, but under "Offensive" under "Strategies." Be aware that it might be difficult for the athlete to name very many strategies.)

- What are the defensive strategies in [sport]? (You are looking for team defensive strategies, such as zone defense versus man-to-man defense in basketball or getting the lead runner out in baseball/softball. Record these as before.)

Feel free to ask whatever questions might get the athlete to tell you what he or she knows. You can give examples, but try not to give so many that the knowledge structure is yours, not the athlete's! You might try other questions first, for example, "How do players score in [sport]?" or "How do you stop the other team from scoring in [sport]?" Even though the suggested interview questions are in an order (skills, then strategies; offense, then defense), you should record information any time an athlete provides it. When the athlete has provided information, you can paraphrase what was said to make sure you understand it. You can also ask, "Are there any others?" This prompts the athlete for more information.

Questions

1. How extensive do you think your athlete's knowledge of the sport is? On what do you base your answer?

2. Did you know more about the sport than your youth athlete, or vice versa? Explain.

3. Did your athlete know more about skills than strategies, an equal amount about each, or more about strategies? Explain.

4. Did your athlete know more about offense or defense? Explain.

5. Do you think you were able to record as much as the athlete knew? If so, how could you tell? If not, why not?

6. Do you think that your athlete's knowledge of this sport would allow him or her to perform at a higher level than would be the case with less knowledge? On what do you base your answer?

Knowledge Structure

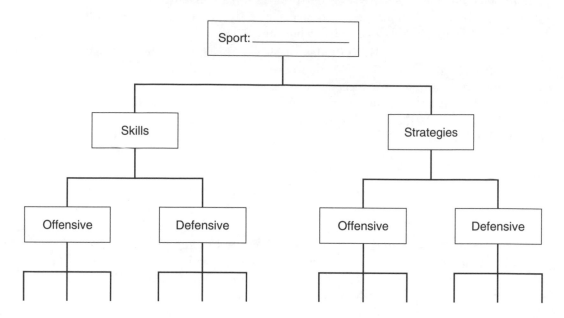

From *Learning Activities for Life Span Motor Development Third Edition* by Kathleen Haywood and Nancy Getchell, 2001, Champaign, IL: Human Kinetics.

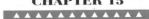

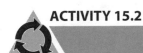 **ACTIVITY 15.2**

Expertise in Senior Athletes

Purpose: To observe the amount of knowledge a senior athlete possesses about his or her sport, especially strategic knowledge.

Many senior athletes have literally decades of experience in their sports or dance forms. As peak physical conditioning declines for many such athletes, they use their experience to compensate with sound, strategic play. In terms of constraints, the functional constraint of knowledge interacts with the structural constraints of strength, flexibility, and so on, as well as with task and environmental constraints. When an individual brings a great deal of knowledge to a context, accomplishment of a goal is possible even as structural constraints limit the movements possible. This was the case with a 58-year-old senior tennis player observed by Langley and Knight (1996). The tennis player was particularly adept at analyzing his opponent's weakness and choosing skills and strategies that took advantage of that weakness.

Sue McPherson and her colleagues have studied sport expertise, including the relationship between knowledge and performance in tennis. In this observation we will use some of her techniques for interviewing a senior tennis player (McPherson, 1999).

Instructions

1. Locate a senior tennis player to interview. This individual should be 55 years or older and should have at least 10 recent years' experience playing competitive tennis. On record sheet 15.2 (p. 179) record the player's gender, age, years of experience in tennis, and any rating or ranking the player holds.

2. Conduct a situation interview with your senior player by asking the three questions listed here. These are three of six questions used by McPherson in previous studies (McPherson, 1999; McPherson & Thomas, 1989). Let your player answer each question as thoroughly as possible. There is no time limit. When the player stops, ask, "Anything else?" until he or she reports there is nothing else to say. These are the questions:

   - What are some of the things you think about before you serve?
   - What are some of the xthings you think about when you are behind the baseline and your opponent is behind the baseline?
   - What are some of the things you think about when you are behind the baseline and your opponent is at the net?

3. Take notes as your senior player is answering each question. You also can audiotape the session if that is acceptable to your interviewee.

4. When you are finished with the third situation, ask your senior player these two questions:

   - Do you have a shot or strategy you have developed as you've gotten older that helps you when playing younger opponents?
   - Do you think your experience helps you when playing younger opponents? How?

5. After your interview, you must analyze the answers given by the senior player. McPherson used a system of first putting parts of the answers to each question in concept categories. We will use four of these categories here:

- Goal concepts: information reflecting how a game is won, the purpose of an action, or the purpose of specifying a condition (e.g., keep the ball in play)
- Condition concepts: information indicating when or under what circumstances actions or patterns of actions are applied to reach a goal
- Action concepts: information about motor or perceptual responses (e.g., hit a forehand down the line, watch for the opponent coming to net)
- Do concepts: information about how to perform or do an action (e.g., "I swing up from below the ball to give it topspin.")

For each part of an answer given by your senior player, briefly enter the part into record sheet 15.2. In the next column indicate whether it is a goal, condition, action, or do concept. For example, let us say your player responded to the first situation by saying that if the opponent had a weak backhand, he or she would serve to the backhand side of the service box. The first part—if the opponent has a weak backhand—is a condition concept because it addresses the circumstances under which the action would be taken. The second part, serving to the backhand, is an action concept because it is information about the response the performer would make. If your player responded that he or she would try to get the service in the service box, this is a goal concept.

6. Finally, for each part of a player's answer, assign the statement a quality level, where Level 1 is an inappropriate or ineffective choice; Level 2 is an appropriate response but the player has no reason for choosing it; and Level 3 is an appropriate response and the player has one or more reasons for choosing it. For example, in responding to the situation in which the player is behind the baseline and the opponent is at the net, the player might say that he or she would simply hit the ball to the opponent in hopes that the opponent would hit it out of bounds; this statement would be Level 1, an ineffective choice. Saying he or she would hit a lob, but without having a reason for doing so, would be Level 2. Saying he or she would hit a lob to move the player back to the baseline would be Level 3. Enter the quality level in the third column of the data table in record sheet 15.2 for each of your entries.

Questions

1. Analyze the amount of information your senior player provided. Was there much information, indicating a rich knowledge of tennis, or was the information limited?

2. Compare and contrast the number of statements that were categorized into each of the four concept categories. McPherson (1999) found that young adult novices in tennis generated more goal-oriented responses whereas young adult experts in tennis generated more condition-oriented responses and more "condition and action" pairs ("If my opponent. . . , then I. . . ."). Did your senior generate relatively more goal-oriented responses or more condition- and action-oriented responses?

3. Analyze the quality levels you assigned to your player's answers. What does this reflect about the level of your player's game? Explain.

4. Did your player have skills or strategies that he or she developed with advancing age to respond to younger and perhaps more conditioned players? Does this seem to agree with your analysis of the situation questions? Explain.

Expertise in Senior Athletes

Interviewee's age _____ Gender _____ Rating/ranking _____

Years of experience in competitive tennis _____

Statement	Concept (goal, condition, action, do)	Quality (1, 2, 3)

From *Learning Activities for Life Span Motor Development Third Edition* by Kathleen Haywood and Nancy Getchell, 2001, Champaign, IL: Human Kinetics.

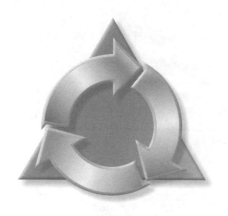

PART VI

Physical Fitness Over the Life Span

CHAPTER 16

Development of Cardiorespiratory Endurance

Of all the aspects of physical fitness, cardiorespiratory endurance is the one considered to have the greatest implications for lifelong health. The adaptations of the circulatory and respiratory systems to repetitive endurance exercise result in a stronger heart muscle and more efficient respiration and circulation.

The benefits of endurance exercise are transitory; that is, it is necessary to exercise appropriately and regularly in order to see improvements in cardiovascular health. If a person stops exercising, cardiovascular health declines. As youths move into adulthood and change their lifestyles, continue into middle adulthood, and then reach older adulthood, it is typical for their activity levels to decline. Cardiovascular health then declines. It is important for people to resist this trend and to participate in regular, appropriate cardiorespiratory endurance exercise throughout life.

The role of exercise in the cardiovascular health of children has been surrounded by several myths over the last century. At one time it was believed that children's cardiovascular and respiratory systems were limited and that prolonged exercise could damage those systems. This myth actually grew from a mismeasurement of children's blood vessel size over 60 years ago! Too, many adults believe that children are active enough in the normal course of their daily lives and that any special efforts to see that children exercise are unnecessary. Today we have increasing evidence that in the age of technology, children can be inactive to the point of being unhealthy.

But children's cardiovascular systems are not just miniature versions of adult's systems; children are undergoing tremendous changes in body size and composition. So, while we know that exercise is beneficial at all ages, it is valuable to study and observe the physiological responses to exercise at each stage of the life span.

ACTIVITY 16.1

Changes in Endurance Performance in Youth

Purpose: To observe changes in cardiorespiratory endurance over a 3-year span of pre-adolescence, noting any gender differences.

There are many forms of cardiorespiratory endurance exercise: running, cycling, swimming, and so on. The body fuels these exercises differently, though, depending on whether the activity is short and intense or long and moderate. During a brief period of intense activity, the body uses local reserves of oxygen and phosphate compounds and breaks down glycogen (energy reserves) to lactic acid. This creates a deficit of oxygen that must be replenished. This process of fueling brief, intense activity is called anaerobic metabolism.

As exercise continues, the anaerobic systems contribute less to fueling the body's movements. Respiration and circulation increase to bring oxygen to the muscles. Chemical changes at the cellular level take over to fuel the working muscles, but these chemical changes can take place only in the presence of oxygen. This process is termed aerobic metabolism. So, prolonged activity is sustained as long as sufficient oxygen can be transported to the working muscles.

An individual's capacity for short, intense activity, or anaerobic activity, is related to body size, especially muscle mass. Since children have less muscle mass than adults have, their anaerobic power is less. As children grow, their muscle mass increases; phosphate concentrations and glycogen content in the muscles increase; tolerance of lactic acid concentrations improves; and consequently anaerobic power increases. Regular participation in anaerobic activities improves anaerobic power in children.

An individual's capacity for prolonged, moderate activity, or aerobic activity, also is related to body size. Aerobic capacity is typically measured by maximal oxygen uptake. Maximal oxygen uptake increases steadily in children, as body size—especially lean body mass—increases. It is interesting that maximal oxygen uptake related to body weight (i.e., when maximal oxygen uptake is divided by body weight) is stable in childhood. There is some question about how much if any benefit children realize from aerobic training, but there is little doubt that training is beneficial once individuals reach puberty.

In this activity, we will analyze children's scores on a test of prolonged, moderate activity, the PACER (Progressive Aerobic Cardiovascular Endurance Run). This test was repeated on 10 children every year for 3 years, beginning at age 10 years, as a part of their school's fitness assessment program.

Instructions

1. Table 16.1 contains the actual scores for five boys and five girls on the PACER of the FITNESSGRAM test battery (Meredith & Welk, 1999). Their physical education teacher shared the scores with us. The FITNESSGRAM is a comprehensive health-related fitness and activity assessment for children. It assesses aerobic capacity; body composition; and muscular strength, endurance, and flexibility. The

PACER is a progressive test of aerobic capacity: it is easy at the beginning and gets progressively harder. In the PACER, children run back and forth between two lines 22 yd (20 m) apart. An audiotape or CD with beeping sounds is played (one version also has music). After a starting signal, children must reach the other line before a beep sounds. They cannot turn to run back to the first line until that beep. The interval between beeps is shortened after each minute. The number of laps, or trips between lines, is counted as the score. Participants continue until the second time they do not reach a line before a beep sounds.

2. Scores for each student's performance on these test items for each of 3 consecutive years are available. Calculate the average score for the boys and girls separately for each year. A space for this is provided in the table. (Recall that an average is obtained by summing all the measures and dividing by the number of measures.)

3. Either by hand on a piece of graph paper, or with a computer software program such as Microsoft® Excel®, plot girls' scores over the 3 years for the PACER. Plot each.individual's scores, and plot the average score. Do the same on another graph for the boys' PACER scores.

Questions

1. Did the PACER scores improve for the boys and for the girls as the children aged? Were these the results you expected? Why or why not?

2. Compare the boys' average and the girls' average, both the actual scores and their respective trends with advancing age. Were they similar or not? Is this what you expected? Why or why not?

3. What physical growth or maturation measurements would be helpful in assessing whether these children are performing consistently with their size or maturation level? If you were the physical education teacher of these children, how would you use these measurements to adjust the goals set for your students?

4. Did every child improve every year? If not, describe a case in which this did not happen. What might account for little or no improvement?

TABLE 16.1			
Changes in Endurance Performance in Youth			
Girls' PACER performance (laps)			
Participant	**Year 1**	**Year 2**	**Year 3**
Girl #1	30	38	48
Girl #2	22	40	46
Girl #3	36	40	46
Girl #4	33	24	46
Girl #5	22	40	46
Group average			

(continued)

TABLE 16.1 *(continued)*

Boys' PACER performance (laps)			
Participant	**Year 1**	**Year 2**	**Year 3**
Boy #1	52	55	76
Boy #2	55	60	75
Boy #3	36	37	50
Boy #4	42	44	42
Boy #5	41	45	76
Group average			

ACTIVITY 16.2

Aerobic and Anaerobic Performance in Older Adulthood

Purpose: To compare age group records for aerobic and anaerobic events and identify trends in performance among older adults.

In the introduction to activity 16.1, we acknowledged that the body fuels brief periods of intense activity differently than it fuels prolonged periods of intense activity. So, events such as the dashes in track and field are fueled differently than longer running events such as the 5,000 and 10,000 m runs. For dashes, the body uses local reserves of oxygen and phosphate compounds and breaks down glycogen (energy reserves) to lactic acid. This type of metabolism is termed *anaerobic*. For longer runs, the body increases respiration and circulation to bring oxygen to the muscles. Oxygen allows chemical changes at the cellular level that can fuel the working muscles for a prolonged period. This type of metabolism is termed *aerobic*.

Both aerobic and anaerobic capacity are related to body size, especially lean body mass. In the general population, older adults tend to lose muscle mass, especially after age 50 years; and the ability to produce and remove lactic acid in the working muscles declines. A decline in anaerobic performance, then, would be expected with advancing age; and at least one study indeed recorded a 50% loss of anaerobic power by age 75 years (Grassi, Cerretelli, Narici, & Marconi, 1991). There has not been very much study of anaerobic power and capacity in older adults who remain active. Reaburn and Mackinnon (1990), though, saw no deterioration in masters athletes who trained for sprint swimming events at the international level.

A decline in aerobic performance also would be expected with advancing age, based on a loss of lean body mass. A decline in the maximum achievable heart rate, as well as a loss of elasticity in the cardiovascular and respiratory tissues, also would contribute to a decline. Indeed, a decline has been documented among athletic, active, and sedentary adults (Spirduso, 1995), although the decline is much smaller among the more active groups. Kasch, Boyer, Van Camp, Verity, & Wallace (1990) observed just a 13% decline in the aerobic capacity of men who maintained training in their 50s and 60s, compared to an average decline of about 40%.

In this exercise, we will examine the age group records established in two short-term and two long-term track events at a regional Senior Olympics. These records were set over a number of years. These data are cross-sectional rather than longitudinal, but nevertheless can provide information about trends in aerobic and anaerobic performance in older adulthood.

Instructions

1. The regional Senior Olympics competitions typically include two track events that can be classified as using anaerobic metabolism, the 50 m dash and the 100 m dash. They also include two track events that can be classified as using aerobic metabolism, the 5,000 m run and the 10,000 m run. The age group records for these four events are presented in table 16.2 for each age group starting with 50- to 54-year-olds and ending with 90- to 94-year-olds. There were no participants in distance events for women past the 75- to 79-year age group or for men past the 85- to 89-year age group. The distance events are presented in terms of minutes and the decimal equivalent of seconds. For example, a record of 18 min 30 sec is presented as 18.5 min.

2. By hand on a piece of graph paper, or with a computer software program such as Microsoft® Excel®, plot four graphs: the women's records for the anaerobic events, the women's records for the aerobic events, the men's records for the anaerobic events, and the men's records for the aerobic events.

TABLE 16.2

Aerobic and Anaerobic Performance in Older Adulthood

Women's records

Event	50-54	55-59	60-64	65-69	70-74	75-79	80-84	85-89	90-94
50 m dash (sec)	8.57	8.16	8.58	8.60	8.77	9.40	9.91	12.31	15.56
100 m dash (sec)	17.64	15.80	16.60	16.40	16.80	18.20	19.49	24.50	32.68
5,000 m run (min)	25.02	23.48	23.52	25.85	29.48	52.80			
10,000 m run (min)	51.18	50.18	48.53	51.52	66.28	68.22			

Men's records

Event	50-54	55-59	60-64	65-69	70-74	75-79	80-84	85-89	90-94
50 m dash (sec)	6.85	6.70	6.59	6.80	7.30	7.90	9.10	9.40	11.02
100 m dash (sec)	12.31	12.14	11.87	12.71	13.48	15.10	17.20	19.60	23.05
5,000 m run (min)	17.52	18.13	18.92	19.92	21.57	24.68	28.23	35.42	
10,000 m run (min)	35.93	37.00	38.10	42.47	44.13	58.78	70.62	67.53	

Questions

1. For each of your four graphs, describe the trend pictured, especially when there are significant changes. At what ages are there notable declines in performance?

2. For men and women separately, compare and contrast the trends pictured for aerobic and anaerobic performance. That is, do changes (declines) occur at the same age or at different ages?

3. From your descriptions and comparsions, what can you conclude about the relationship between aerobic and anaerobic performance? On what do you base your conclusions?

4. Were you surprised that the 50- to 54-year-old group was not always the best? Why or why not? It might help to know that this age group was only recently added to the competition. How might this influence performance records? What other factors might influence them?

CHAPTER 17

Development of Strength and Flexibility

The course of development differs for muscular strength and musculoskeletal flexibility. Strength is linked to the development of muscle mass, although increases in strength do not always parallel increases in muscle mass. Recall from your textbook that muscle mass follows a sigmoid growth pattern. Gender differences are minimal until puberty, when boys add significantly more muscle mass than girls do, especially in the upper body. From young adulthood until the age of 50 there is small loss of muscle, but thereafter the loss can be pronounced. This older adult trend is related to activity level and nutrition.

Muscle mass, though, is not the only factor in strength. The force exerted by a muscle depends on both the cross-sectional size of the muscle and the degree of coordination in activating the muscle fibers. The importance of the latter neurologic factors is illustrated by the fact that during adolescence, the peak velocity for increases in strength occurs slightly later than the peak velocity for increases in muscle mass. So, increases in muscle mass and in strength are not always parallel, but in general there is improvement in strength throughout childhood and adolescence.

The same is not necessarily true for flexibility. Flexibility is the ability to move joints through a full range of motion. Exercise and training, either through a systematic flexibility program or through participation in physical activities, can involve some joints more than others. Individuals can have acceptable flexibility in some joints while having limited range of motion in others, putting the muscle surrounding the latter at risk of injury or limiting peak performance. Flexibility truly follows the "use it or lose it" phenomenon in fitness training.

Infants and toddlers are obviously very flexible, so it is easy for parents, teachers, and coaches to overlook the importance of flexibility exercise for children. Research studies have tended to show, though, that children and adolescents can lose flexibility in joints not exercised as they grow and develop. This trend continues throughout the life span and becomes significant after age 49. Extreme losses of flexibility in older adulthood can limit the activities of daily living.

Both strength and flexibility are influenced, then, by the extent of training to maintain or increase strength and flexibility. In the following activities we will observe strength or flexibility and then discuss the results of our observations in light of individuals' training programs. We will use data provided to us by an elementary school that uses the FITNESSGRAM assessment and reporting system (Meredith & Welk, 1999). The FITNESSGRAM is a comprehensive health-related fitness and activity assessment for children. It assesses aerobic capacity; body composition; and muscular strength, endurance, and flexibility.

ACTIVITY 17.1

Examining Trends in Strength Development

Purpose: To observe changes in functional strength in preadolescence, noting gender differences and body area differences.

Strength can vary within an individual in various body areas. Muscle mass can be relatively greater or smaller in different body areas. These differences are related to genetic predispositions and the level of training or participation in strength-building activities one undertakes. So, getting a truly accurate picture of how strong a person is requires assessment of the various body areas.

Of course, such an exhaustive assessment is impractical in some situations. Fitness tests conducted in the schools typically are done during physical education classes, and time is limited. Those who design such assessments often choose a few tests of strength to represent overall strength. Moreover, these assessments are usually functional measures. That is, they are measurements that can be obtained with minimal equipment. A researcher in a laboratory setting would probably use equipment to measure the force one could exert during movement at a variety of joints, in a variety of directions, and possibly at a variety of speeds. Teachers and coaches are more likely to measure the number of repetitions one can complete in moving the body weight against the resistance of gravity, or the length of time one can support body weight.

The FITNESSGRAM assessment uses representative functional measurements of strength. Teachers can choose among several tests. The teachers who provided the scores we are using here chose curl-ups (see figure 17.1, a and b), as a measure of abdominal strength and muscle endurance; the flexed-arm hang (see figure 17.2), as a measure of upper body strength and endurance; and the trunk lift (see figure 17.3, a and b, on p. 190), as a measure of trunk extensor strength and flexibility. In the curl-up assessment, children are asked to complete as many curl-ups as possible, up to a maximum of 75, at a specified pace that is called by the teacher or played from an audio tape or CD (a pace of approximately 20 curl-ups per minute). The distance of the "curl" is controlled by having the children lie on their backs and move their arms along the mat as they curl up, their fingertips traveling a specified distance along the mat. An individual continues until 75 curl-ups have been performed or a second form correction is made. Corrections are made for bringing the heels off the mat, not returning the head to the mat on every repetition, pausing or resting, and not reaching the target location with the fingertips.

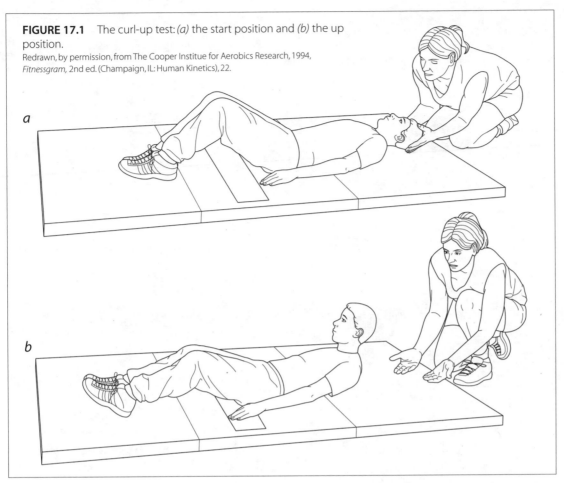

FIGURE 17.1 The curl-up test: (a) the start position and (b) the up position.
Redrawn, by permission, from The Cooper Institue for Aerobics Research, 1994, *Fitnessgram,* 2nd ed. (Champaign, IL: Human Kinetics), 22.

a

b

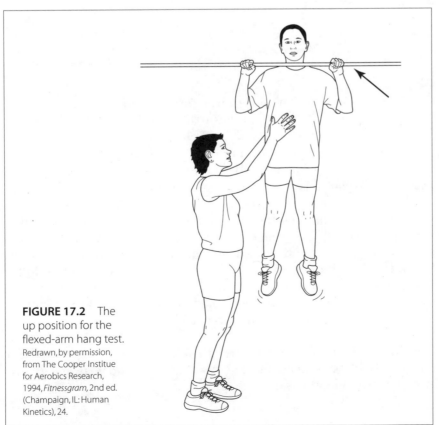

FIGURE 17.2 The up position for the flexed-arm hang test.
Redrawn, by permission, from The Cooper Institue for Aerobics Research, 1994, *Fitnessgram,* 2nd ed. (Champaign, IL: Human Kinetics), 24.

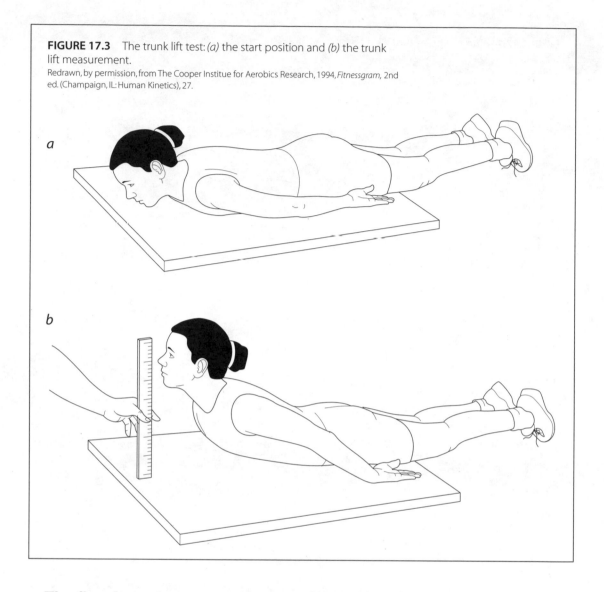

FIGURE 17.3   The trunk lift test: *(a)* the start position and *(b)* the trunk lift measurement.
Redrawn, by permission, from The Cooper Institue for Aerobics Research, 1994, *Fitnessgram,* 2nd ed. (Champaign, IL: Human Kinetics), 27.

a

b

The flexed-arm hang uses a horizontal bar. Children grasp the bar with an overhand grip. A spotter helps them raise their bodies off the floor so that their chins are above the bar, elbows flexed, and chests close to the bar. A stopwatch is started as soon as they are in position and stopped when the chin touches the bar, the head tilts back to keep the chin above the bar, or the chin falls below the level of the bar. Children can have one form correction; a second correction ends the test.

In the trunk lift test, children lie prone on a mat, toes pointed and hands placed under the thighs. A marker is placed on the floor in line with the students' eyes. Students maintain focus on this marker throughout. Children slowly lift their bodies off the floor, to a maximum height of 12 in. (30 cm). They hold the position just long enough for an observer to place a ruler in front of them and note the distance between the mat and the chin. The best score of two trials is allowed. The maximum score discourages excessive arching that may compress the spinal discs.

It is interesting to observe changes in strength as preadolescents proceed through their growth period. We will focus on change in boys as a group and girls as a group, as well as patterns of change in individuals.

Instructions

1. Table 17.1 contains the scores for five boys and five girls on the three items of the FITNESSGRAM test battery we have described. Scores are available for each student's performance on these test items for each of 3 consecutive years. Calculate the average score for the boys and girls separately for each year for each test item. A space for this is provided in the table. (Recall that an average is obtained by summing all the measures and dividing by the number of measures.)

2. Either by hand on a piece of graph paper or with a computer software program such as Microsoft® Excel®, plot girls' scores over the 3 years for curl-ups. Plot each individual's score and plot the average score. Do the same on another graph for the boys' curl-up scores.

3. Again by hand or with a software program, plot girls' scores over the 3 years for the flexed-arm hang. Plot each individual's scores and plot the average score. Do the same on another graph for the boys' flexed-arm hang scores.

4. Finally, plot the girls' trunk lift distance over the 3 years. Plot each individual at each year as well as the average distance for the group. Do the same for the boys on another graph.

Questions

1. Focusing on your plots of the group averages, did the boys and girls get stronger with age? Was their improvement linear, that is, did it increase approximately the same amount each year? Or were there years of greater and lesser improvement? Is this what you would expect from what we know of developmental trends in strength? Why or why not? Are your answers to these questions the same for abdominal and for upper body strength, or were there differences?

2. How did the boys as a group compare to the girls as a group on curl-up performance? On flexed-arm hang? On trunk lift distance? Do these two groups follow the typical gender differences in strength between boys and girls of this age?

3. Now focus your attention on the individuals' scores. Did individuals tend to follow the same pattern of improvement as the group average (that is, did some remain above average over the 3 years, some remain average, and some remain below average)? Or, did some "change places" within the group? (Another way of examining this is to observe whether individuals maintained their place in the group over the 3 years. For example, was the strongest individual in Year 1 the strongest in Years 2 and 3?) If some individuals changed places, what could account for this? (Consider both internal and external factors.)

4. Again focusing on individuals, were the same boys and girls the strongest or weakest on both the abdominal and upper body assessments? Or did you find individuals who were strong in one area but weaker in the other? Describe any such cases.

5. Note that the flexed-arm hang uses body weight for resistance. How would an increase in fat weight affect performance on these particular measurements? Would boys or girls be more likely to add fat weight over this age period?

TABLE 17.1

Examining Trends in Strength Development

Girls' curl-up performance

Participant	Year 1	Year 2	Year 3
Girl #1	30	37	34
Girl #2	21	22	44
Girl #3	30	27	29
Girl #4	21	31	31
Girl #5	25	42	34
Group average			

Boys' curl-up performance

Participant	Year 1	Year 2	Year 3
Boy #1	23	30	20
Boy #2	19	19	34
Boy #3	30	39	33
Boy #4	25	25	30
Boy #5	30	22	33
Group average			

Girls' flexed-arm hang performance (sec)

Participant	Year 1	Year 2	Year 3
Girl #1	6.8	18.0	18.8
Girl #2	8.5	10.0	25.9
Girl #3	14.0	9.0	20.8
Girl #4	6.0	11.0	22.3
Girl #5	2.4	4.5	7.6
Group average			

Boys' flexed-arm hang performance (sec)			
Participant	Year 1	Year 2	Year 3
Boy #1	31.0	31.0	48.0
Boy #2	6.2	7.0	8.0
Boy #3	7.0	8.0	6.6
Boy #4	3.6	4.1	10.4
Boy #5	4.4	6.6	20.8
Group average			

Girls' trunk lift (in.; 12 in. [30 cm] maximum)			
Participant	Year 1	Year 2	Year 3
Girl #1	12	12	10
Girl #2	12	12	12
Girl #3	11	12	12
Girl #4	10	11	9
Girl #5	12	12	12
Group average			

Boys' trunk lift (in.; 12 in. [30 cm] maximum)			
Participant	Year 1	Year 2	Year 3
Boy #1	11	12	12
Boy #2	10	8	12
Boy #3	12	12	12
Boy #4	12	12	12
Boy #5	12	12	12
Group average			

▲ **ACTIVITY 17.2**

Examining Trends in Sit-and-Reach Performance

Purpose: To observe changes in sit-and-reach performance, as a representative assessment of flexibility, in preadolescence.

As we mentioned earlier, one's degree of flexibility is specific to joints. A complete flexibility assessment would require testing of each of the body's major joints and of both the left and right sides of the body. Obviously, test batteries must often select a small number of measurements to keep the length of testing short and practical. In many youth fitness test batteries the sit-and-reach test is the representative flexibility measurement. When youth fitness assessments were designed initially, the sit-and-reach test was chosen as a spine and hip flexibility measurement. Low back pain was known to be a major health concern, and a lack of flexibility was hypothesized as a contributing factor.

Use of the sit-and-reach test in fitness batteries has demonstrated somewhat stable performance between ages 6 and 9 years (Ross, Pate, Delpy, Gold, & Svilar, 1987). Thereafter, boys improve their sit-and-reach scores (Beunen, Malina, Renson, & Van Gerven, 1988). Girls are stable until approximately age 12 years; then girls in the upper percentiles improve whereas those in the lower percentiles decline (Simons et al., 1990).

The sit-and-reach test presents several concerns for researchers and teachers who use it. First, sit-and-reach flexibility is measured relative to a point even with the feet. A small number of individuals with unusually long legs, short arms, or both are placed at a disadvantage in the test. Second, those who abduct the shoulder blades increase their score as compared with those who do not. Finally, abdominal *strength* might play a role in the improvement in scores in adolescence. That is, individuals with strong abdominal muscles can pull the trunk forward to a greater degree of flexion. So, it is important to realize that exercise and training, both for strength and for range of motion, can contribute to sit-and-reach performance.

In this activity you will use data from the same group of students as in activity 17.1. These students performed the back-saver sit-and-reach item, an optional assessment in the FITNESSGRAM (see figure 17.4). The back-saver sit and reach is similar to the traditional sit and reach, but only one leg is extended against the sit-and-reach box while the other is bent, with the sole of the foot flat on the floor. This makes it less likely that children will hurt their lower backs.

FIGURE 17.4 The back-saver sit and reach with only the right leg extended against the box.
Redrawn, by permission, from The Cooper Institue for Aerobics Research, 1994, *Fitnessgram*, 2nd ed. (Champaign, IL: Human Kinetics), 29.

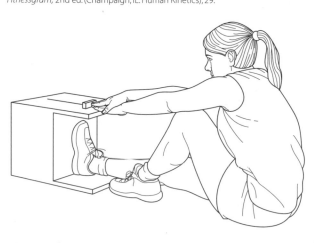

Instructions

1. Table 17.2 contains the scores for five boys and five girls on the sit-and-reach item of the FITNESSGRAM test battery. Scores are available for each student's performance on these test items for each of 3 consecutive years. Calculate the average score for the boys and girls separately for each year. A space for this is provided in the table. (Recall that an average is obtained by summing all the measures and dividing by the number of measures.)

2. Either by hand on a piece of graph paper, or with a computer software program, such as Microsoft® Excel®, plot girls' scores over the 3 years for sit-and-reach performance. Plot each individual's scores and plot the average score. Do the same on another graph for the boys' scores.

Questions

1. Focusing first on your plot of the group averages, did the boys and girls increase or decrease in flexibility with advancing age? Was the trend linear; that is, did it change the same amount from year to year? Or were there years of greater or lesser change? Is this what you expected from what we know of developmental trends in sit-and-reach performance?

2. Now focus on individuals. Did individuals tend to maintain their place within the group over the 3 years? That is, did the most flexible child remain the most flexible and the least flexible remain the least flexible? If not, to what would you attribute this finding?

3. How did the boys as a group and the girls as a group compare? Is this what you expected? Why or why not?

4. If you completed activity 17.1, compare the flexibility scores in this activity with the strength scores in activity 17.1 (Boy #1 is the same in both learning activities, Girl #1 the same, etc.). Are the same children the strongest and most flexible or the weakest and least flexible? Is this what you would have expected? Why or why not?

TABLE 17.2

Examining Trends in Sit-and-Reach Performance			
Girls' sit-and-reach scores (in.)			
Participant	**Year 1**	**Year 2**	**Year 3**
Girl #1	9	13	15
Girl #2	15	15	15
Girl #3	15	14	14
Girl #4	12	10	12
Girl #5	11	12	13
Group average			
Boys' sit-and-reach scores (in.)			
Participant	**Year 1**	**Year 2**	**Year 3**
Boy #1	10	10	10
Boy #2	10	8	11
Boy #3	11	10	10
Boy #4	12	10	10
Boy #5	10	10	12
Group average			

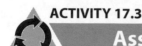

ACTIVITY 17.3

Assessing Flexibility in Older Adulthood

Purpose: To observe the flexibility of a middle-aged or older adult and to relate that degree of flexibility to the extent and type of the individual's physical activity.

Range of movement in the joints, or flexibility, is determined by elasticity of the body tissues. Unfortunately, inactivity works against elasticity. Most people aren't aware of gradually losing this elasticity until they realize in middle or late adulthood that they can't move the way they once could. Without a systematic exercise program to maintain and promote flexibility, range of motion begins to shrink in childhood and continues to do so over one's life span.

Repetitious movements, carried out over years and years, also are problematic. These movements can shorten the musculature on one side of a joint while making the opposing side lax. The result can be a loss of range of motion in some plane of movement and even overuse injury.

You will have the opportunity in this activity to check the flexibility of a middle-aged or older adult. You will use several simple tests that should not leave your subject sore or stiff. Answers of "no" on the test items indicate that the individual has lost flexibility to an extent that affects body function.

Instructions

1. Work with an adult over 50 years of age. Before administering the test, familiarize yourself with the test items so that you can explain them. Now ask your adult to do each of the test items.

2. Record your results on record sheet 17.1.

3. Ask about any exercise programs in which the individual participates, as well as any sport or dance activities done regularly and any tasks at home or work that are physical and/or repetitious. Make notes on this interview at the bottom of the record sheet.

Questions

1. Has your subject lost flexibility to an extent that body function is affected? Cite results to support your answer. Does this agree with the activity level your adult reported?

2. Did your subject pass or fail the four tests? Flexibility can vary from joint to joint in an individual. Did you find this to be the case with your subject? Do your results match up with the activities reported by your subject? That is, did she or he report an activity involving a body area that your test showed had good flexibility?

3. Was your subject equally flexible in the right and left arms and shoulders? Is this what you expected? Why or why not? Did your subject report any activity that would account for equal or unequal flexibility?

Assessing Flexibility in Older Adulthood

Adult's age _____ Adult's sex _____ Adult's birth date _____

Test item	Result	
1. Have your subject sit on the floor with the back against a wall. Direct the subject to stretch one leg out in front then draw the foot of the other leg up against the thigh. Is the knee of the extended leg flat against the floor?	Yes	No
2. Direct your subject to raise arms overhead, fingertips pointing to the ceiling. Are the arms even with or behind the ears?	Yes	No
Are the arms equally flexible?	Yes	No
3. Have your subject stand facing you, arms at sides. Direct the subject to turn hands outward without moving the elbows away from the body. Can you see the palms?	Yes	No
Are the palms equally visible?	Yes	No
4. Direct your subject to stand, to place arms behind the back and link hands, then to pull the hands away from the back. Are the hands raised to a level even with the waist?	Yes	No

Notes

From *Learning Activities for Life Span Motor Development Third Edition* by Kathleen Haywood and Nancy Getchell, 2001, Champaign, IL: Human Kinetics.

Assessments based on *The rejuvenation strategy: A medically approved fitness program to reverse the effects of aging* by R. Cailliet and L. Gross, 1987 (Garden City, NY: Doubleday).

CHAPTER 18

Development of Body Composition

In the context of physical growth and aging and motor development, body composition refers to the relative composition of the body in terms of fat or adipose tissue and lean body mass (muscles, bones, and organs). Monitoring body composition is important in preventing obesity. Obesity is associated with a greater risk of several aspects of poor health, especially coronary heart disease, stroke, and diabetes. Unfortunately, the trend is toward increased incidence of obesity at all ages, including childhood. Beyond an association with good health, a body composition lower in fat tissue and higher in muscle tissue is associated with good performance in a variety of physical activities.

Those interested in motor development, then, have a dual purpose in attending to the interaction between exercise or physical activity and one's body composition. Physical activities tend to burn calories and reduce the amount of fat while promoting muscle development. For good health and wellness, regular exercise at any age helps to maintain a desirable body composition. Even those who are not interested in sport or dance performance need regular exercise. For those who are interested in optimal sport and dance performance, exercise to decrease fat weight (as long as this is not carried to an extreme) and increase muscle weight is necessary. Both genetic and extrinsic factors impact body composition. It is the extrinsic factors of diet and exercise that individuals can use to influence their body composition.

We know that the general trends are for fat tissue to increase shortly after birth and again in adolescence, especially in girls. Muscle tissue grows rapidly in infancy, steadily in childhood, and again rapidly in adolescence, especially in boys. Beginning even in young adulthood there is a trend toward increased fat weight, and then in older adulthood a trend toward decreased muscle weight. So, body composition changes over the life span. Through diet and exercise, individuals can influence the extent to which they follow these trends. The effects, of course, are transient. To achieve a positive effect on body composition, one must maintain a healthy diet and exercise program throughout life!

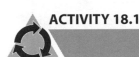

ACTIVITY 18.1

Body Composition in Childhood

Purpose: To follow changes in body mass index (BMI) in a group of children over a period of 4.0 years.

Following body composition in childhood has at least two positive effects. First, the trend is toward increased fatness among children today. Attention to body composition can avoid the onset of obesity in childhood, a health concern that is difficult to reverse later in life. Second, attention to body composition can teach children about healthy levels of fat and muscle and establish behavioral patterns to help them maintain that healthy level throughout their lives. Most physical fitness test batteries for children include a measure or estimate of body composition.

There are many methods of measuring body composition in children, including underwater weighing, skinfold measurement, bioelectrical impedance, and BMIs based on height and weight. Each has advantages and disadvantages, and each has limitations that lead to measurement errors. These measurement errors typically are in the range of 2 to 3%, but can be as high as 5 to 6% for estimates based on height and weight. The most practical measurements for school programs are skinfold thickness in the upper arm and calf and BMI based on height and weight.

In this activity, we will use the BMI measures taken on five boys and five girls as part of the regular physical fitness testing in their physical education program. We have measurements taken every fall and spring from the age of approximately 5.5 years to 9.5 years. We will be able to look at change over a substantial part of the childhood period.

Instructions

1. Body mass index for five boys and five girls from age 5.5 years to 9.5 years is presented on record sheet 18.1 (p. 201). Calculate the average BMI for the girls, then for the boys, at each age of measurement. Enter these values on record sheet 18.1. (Recall that an average is calculated by summing scores and then dividing by the number of scores summed.)

2. Using a computer software program, such as Microsoft® Excel® or by hand on graph paper, graph the BMI over the nine measurement times for each of the five girls and the average for the girls.

3. Do the same for the boys.

Questions

1. Look at your graph of the girls' measures. Is there a trend toward an increased or decreased BMI for the individual girls or for the group average? What about the individual boys or their group average? On what do you base your answers?

2. Consult the United States National Center for Health Statistics graph of body mass index-for-age percentiles, ages 2 to 20 years, both for boys and for girls (available in appendix B [figure B.2, a and b]). Compare the data for the boys and girls in this activity to the percentiles plotted on the charts. Generally, are these boys and girls at the higher percentiles, at the lower percentiles, or around the 50th percentile? Explain your answers.

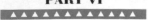
3. Consider Boy #4 and Girl #2. The changes in their heights and weights over the 5.5 years, along with their BMIs, are shown in table 18.1. Examine the changes in height and weight. Do increases in height, weight, or both seem to change the BMI? Explain your answer.

TABLE 18.1

Boy #4									
	5.5	**6.0**	**6.5**	**7.0**	**7.5**	**8.0**	**8.5**	**9.0**	**9.5**
Ht (ft, in)	4'1"	4'2"	4'4"	4'5"	4'6"	4'7"	4'8"	4'10"	4'11"
Wt (lbs)	60	66	71	76	79	85	95	97	104
BMI	17.6	18.6	18.4	19.0	19.0	19.7	21.3	20.3	21.0

Girl #2									
	5.5	**6.0**	**6.5**	**7.0**	**7.5**	**8.0**	**8.5**	**9.0**	**9.5**
Ht (ft, in)	3'9"	3'11"	4'0"	4'1"	4'3"	4'3"	4'4"	4'5"	4'7"
Wt (lbs)	43	57	67	73	73	76	81	91	98
BMI	14.9	18.1	20.4	21.4	19.7	20.5	21.1	22.9	22.8

Body Composition in Childhood

Age	5.5	6.0	6.5	7.0	7.5	8.0	8.5	9.0	9.5
Girl #1	14.0	14.9	15.2	15.8	15.4	16.5	16.0	16.7	16.8
Girl #2	14.9	18.1	20.4	21.4	19.7	20.5	21.1	22.9	22.8
Girl #3	14.3	13.8	13.8	14.3	14.0	14.2	14.2	13.8	14.4
Girl #4	14.6	14.0	14.0	14.0	13.5	14.3	14.0	13.8	14.0
Girl #5	14.9	14.6	15.5	16.4	16.0	15.6	16.8	*	*
Girls' avg.									
Boy #1	17.2	17.7	*	19.1	19.2	19.5	19.3	20.0	18.8
Boy #2	15.9	15.7	15.6	16.4	15.4	15.7	16.5	15.8	15.3
Boy #3	13.0	13.9	13.4	14.0	13.0	13.5	14.0	13.3	13.5
Boy #4	17.6	18.6	18.4	19.0	19.0	19.7	21.3	20.3	21.0
Boy #5	*	15.5	14.6	15.1	14.0	14.9	15.0	15.6	15.9
Boys' avg.									

*Student was not measured.

From *Learning Activities for Life Span Motor Development Third Edition* by Kathleen Haywood and Nancy Getchell, 2001, Champaign, IL: Human Kinetics.

ACTIVITY 18.2

Comparing Body Composition Measures

Purpose: To compare a body composition measure based on skinfold thickness to one based on height and weight.

There are several ways to measure body composition. Underwater weighing and bio-electrical impedance measures require equipment, and schools or senior exercise programs rarely have this equipment available. Skinfold measures require a set of calipers. Although calipers can be very expensive, there are several plastic types that are not expensive and are easy to obtain. The person taking the measure, though, must be familiar with the appropriate technique and must be careful to take the measure at the correct location. Body mass index is probably the easiest measure to obtain, since it is simply an individual's weight in kilograms divided by the square of his or her height in meters.

Measurement error is a concern for all these measures, but in particular for BMI, since the measurement error associated with two separate measures, height and weight, can compound, leading to a total measurement error of 5 to 6%. That is, the true value might be 5 to 6% higher or lower than the obtained value.

In addition, since BMI is based in part on body weight, this ratio tends to treat individuals with a higher portion of fat weight and those with a higher portion of muscle weight as if they were the same. That is, scale weight does not distinguish between "heaviness" due to excess fat weight and that due to additional muscle weight. Estimates of percent fat based on skinfold measures should avoid this problem, but they have the additional problem of reflecting subcutaneous fat at the particular sites on the body where the thicknesses are measured. We know that the deposit of subcutaneous fat tends to change over the life span. Subcutaneous fat is small until age 6 or 7 years, then increases. It plateaus or actually decreases in boys after age 12 to 13, but can continue to increase in girls. The subcutaneous fat that boys add after age 13 tends to be on the trunk more than on the limbs, whereas girls add subcutaneous fat in both locations. Moving from adulthood to older adulthood, individuals tend to add subcutaneous fat to the trunk if they increase their fat weight. Researchers have generated various formulas to estimate percent fat from skinfold measures to reflect the likely distribution of fat at certain ages and to reflect gender differences. Individuals, though, can differ from the typical pattern, and thus a particular formula can do a better or poorer job of estimating their actual percent fat.

In this activity, you will select several individuals and determine a body composition measure based on skinfold thickness as well as one based on height and weight. You then will examine how truly reflective of the individual the two measures appear to be.

Equipment List

Skinfold calipers

Scale

Stadiometer or tape measure mounted on the wall

Instructions

1. Locate eight individuals representing various points of the life span from child-hood to older adulthood.

2. Measure each person's height and weight. Use the methods described in activity 3.2 (p. 26). If you take your measurements in English units, convert them to metric measures. Additionally, convert height measurement in centimeters to meters. Calculate the BMI for each individual by dividing the person's weight in kilograms by the square of the person's height in meters; or use the chart in appendix B to read the BMI directly, based on the individual's height and weight. Record your values on record sheet 18.2 (p. 206).

3. For children or pubescent youths, measure skinfold thickness at the triceps site and the calf site as described in activity 3.2 (p. 27). Estimate each child's percent fat using the method described on p. 28 (sum the two skinfold measures).

4. For adult women, measure skinfold thickness at the triceps site as described in activity 3.2, as well as the suprailiac site (see figure 18.1). To find the suprailiac site, in the general area of the waist in the front of the body, feel for the iliac (pelvic bone) crest. The fold should be taken just above the iliac crest in line with the natural angle of the crest (diagonal to absolute horizontal; see figure 18.1). Use figure 18.2 to estimate the percent fat for each woman. Mark the triceps skinfold value measured on the left vertical line and the suprailiac skinfold value measured on the right vertical line. Connect the two marks with a straight line. The estimated percent fat is the value where that line crosses the middle vertical scale.

5. For adult men, measure skinfold thickness at the subscapular site and the thigh site (see figures 18.3 and 18.4). To find the subscapular site, feel for the lower tip of the scapula. The fold should be a diagonal one, at 45° up and in, taken 0.8 in. (2 cm) below the lower tip of the scapula. To find the thigh site, find the point half

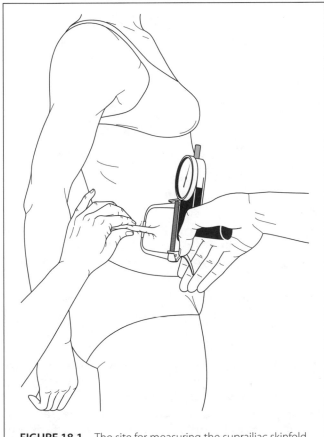

FIGURE 18.1   The site for measuring the suprailiac skinfold.

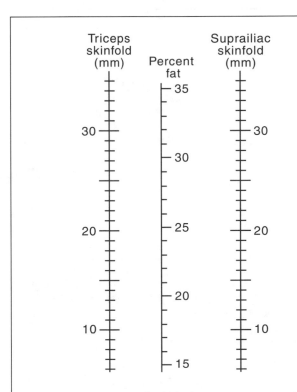

FIGURE 18.2   Percent body fat for women estimated from the triceps and suprailiac skinfolds.

From *Your guide to getting fit*, third edition, by Ivan Kusinitz and Morton Fine. Copyright © 1995 by Mayfield Publishing Company. Reprinted by permission of the publisher.

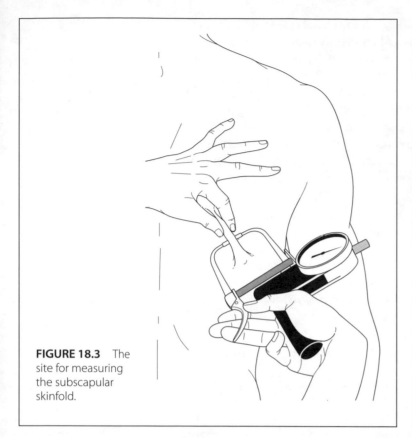

FIGURE 18.3   The site for measuring the subscapular skinfold.

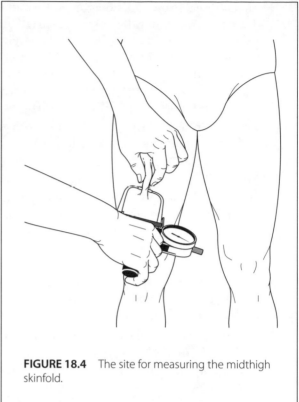

FIGURE 18.4   The site for measuring the midthigh skinfold.

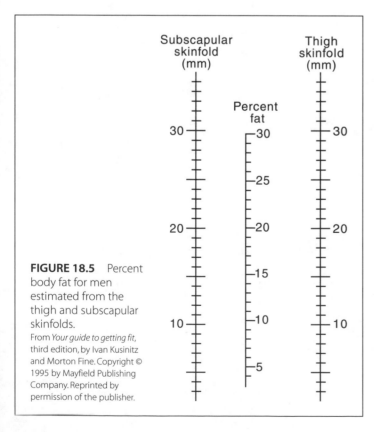

FIGURE 18.5   Percent body fat for men estimated from the thigh and subscapular skinfolds.

From *Your guide to getting fit*, third edition, by Ivan Kusinitz and Morton Fine. Copyright © 1995 by Mayfield Publishing Company. Reprinted by permission of the publisher.

the distance between the top of the kneecap and the leg/trunk crease. The fold should be on the midline of the thigh. Use figure 18.5 to estimate the percent fat for each man using the same method as already described for women.

Questions

1. Using table 18.2 for the adults and appendix A for the children, determine the category into which each of your individuals falls based on skinfold measures: very low fat, low fat, optimal range, moderately high fat, high fat, or very high fat. Now, use appendix B (table B.1) to determine the category into which each person would fall based on BMI.

2. How many of your individuals are in the optimal range? How many are lower than the optimal range? How many are higher? Are there any individuals who fall into one category based on skinfold measures but another based on BMI? Describe their cases. (Note: There are six categories based on skinfold and only four based on BMI, but for the purpose of the comparison you can combine "very low fat" and "low fat" and combine "moderately high fat" and "high fat.")

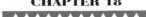

3. Think about the eight individuals you measured. Do you think that one or the other measurement method over- or underestimated any individual's percent fat? Why do you think so?

4. Based on your activities and findings here, what measurement method do you prefer? Why?

TABLE 18.2

Interpreting Body Fat Percentages		
Category	**Men (% fat)**	**Women (% fat)**
Very low fat	< 10	< 17
Low fat	10-12	17-19
Optimal range	13-16	20-24
Moderately high fat	17-19	25-29
High fat	20-24	30-34
Very high fat	> 24	> 34

Comparing Body Composition Measures

	Gender	Age	Height	Weight	BMI	Skinfolds	% fat
#1			English: Metric:	English: Metric:		#1 #2	
#2			English: Metric:	English: Metric:		#1 #2	
#3			English: Metric:	English: Metric:		#1 #2	
#4			English: Metric:	English: Metric:		#1 #2	
#5			English: Metric:	English: Metric:		#1 #2	
#6			English: Metric:	English: Metric:		#1 #2	
#7			English: Metric:	English: Metric:		#1 #2	
#8			English: Metric:	English: Metric:		#1 #2	

From *Learning Activities for Life Span Motor Development Third Edition* by Kathleen Haywood and Nancy Getchell, 2001, Champaign, IL: Human Kinetics.

CHAPTER 19

Interactions Among Individual, Environmental, and Task Constraints

To this point in *Learning Activities for Life Span Motor Development,* we have emphasized that various types of constraints affect motor development and that the influence of any constraint changes across the life span. In order to conceptualize how constraints work, we have separated them into individual, environmental, and task. Remember, however, that although one type of constraint may have more influence, all constraints exist and constantly interact at any given time. In a practical sense, constraints do not exist without individuals' moving in a context. That means that you must understand how the interaction of constraints *constructs* movement. This may seem a difficult task at first! However, assessing the influence of constraints on one another is what we have been doing all along. Remember our example in chapter 3 of the textbook about the young man who was recruited as early as his freshman year to play basketball? The significance of the story is related to his individual constraints (height, strength), environmental constraints (availability of courts, sociocultural expectation of playing basketball), and task constraints (rules of basketball, size of ball) all acting together.

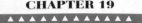
If any of the constraints had been different, his motor development would have been different. For example, what if he grew up in Sweden, where basketball is not as popular a sport as it is in other countries?

You can better understand motor development in a practical way by analyzing the influence of various constraints. Then, you can use this information to help you as a movement specialist; you can manipulate different constraints to allow different behaviors to come forth. We would like to emphasize this point: If a change in a constraint leads to a change in the interaction between constraints, then it can lead to a change in motor behavior. In other words, we can influence our own motor behavior and that of others. Isn't that the point of teaching and rehabilitation?

ACTIVITY 19.1

Making Decisions About Constraints Within a Real-World Movement Context

Purpose: To identify the influence of different constraints acting within a movement context and to make decisions based on these identifications.

The first few times you attempt it, you may have difficulty in determining the relative influence of different types of constraints in movement contexts. Like any skill, it takes practice. This learning activity is designed to provide you with this practice in a problem-solving situation. You will critically read a movement scenario, make decisions about the relevant constraints and how they interact, and then make decisions on what you could do or advise in this scenario in order to change the interaction of constraints and thereby influence movement behavior.

Instructions

For each of the following scenarios, you will do the following:

1. Read the scenario completely.
2. Identify the most important constraints that act in this scenario.
3. Locate information from the text or other sources about these constraints.
4. Make an informed decision on what you could do or advise that would modify or change the emergent motor behavior.

Make sure that you provide rationales that are based on research or a valid information source rather than simply your own opinion. Remember to reference your sources, even if it is just to note the page where you found the information in the text.

> **Scenario I**
>
> You teach movement activities at a local middle school. Your colleague has spearheaded a proposal to have single-sex physical education classes for boys and girls. The school board comes to you, with your expansive knowledge of motor development, to comment on this proposal and make recommendations. What is your position and why?

Scenario II

Your neighbor is a 67-year-old widower. He has mild arthritis and cataracts. He has not exercised consistently in 30 years, but he would like to begin an exercise program and asks you for some advice. What can you tell him about aging and physical fitness in general and about what he should do specifically?

Scenario III

You teach a physical education class of 20 first graders in an urban school. Within your class, you have two students with disabilities—a boy with ADHD (attention deficit hyperactivity disorder) and a girl with visual impairments. Provide a general developmental profile of first-grade children. What types of activities should you teach in class and why? How can you modify these activities to fully include the students with disabilities?

Scenario IV

Consider your own motor development across your life span. What constraints have influenced your motor behavior the most? Remember to consider all classifications of constraints. How have these constraints changed since you were a child? How might these change in the future?

ACTIVITY 19.2

Determining Constraints in a Practical Setting

Purpose: To identify constraints in a real-world movement setting.

The information and exercises provided in the third edition of *Life Span Motor Development*, along with the learning activities in this guide, have culminated to this point. You should now be able to identify the critical constraints interacting in a context, then make informed decisions about how to change that interaction to allow desired motor behaviors to emerge. You will explore a real-world context and try to determine types of constraints as well as their interactions. You will then use this information to problem solve and make decisions about changing interactions to allow motor behaviors to emerge. These skills will help you to become a better observer and practitioner, regardless of your field of interest.

Instructions

1. Pick a movement context that is of interest to you. For example, if you are interested in elementary school physical education, you might pick a second-grade physical education class. If you are interested in gerontology, you might pick an older adult fitness class. Your instructor may have a specific context in which he or she would like you to observe.

2. Plan to spend a full practice or activity period observing movement within this context. Often, staff in schools or programs are happy to allow you to watch, as long as you give them plenty of prior notice of your coming.

3. When you arrive at the location you are to observe, make a detailed check of the environment. What are the most important features of the environment? What are subtle features that affect movement? Describe the environment in detail.

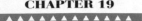
4. Next, look at the group as a whole. What are the general characteristics of the group?

5. Detail what the task is. Include specific information wherever possible. For example, don't write "dribble a basketball," but include rules about double dribbling.

6. Next, pick out two individuals within this particular environment. Try to choose people who appear to have different individual constraints. Describe the results of the individuals' performance of a task within the environment. Compare and contrast the two individuals, focusing on how the differing interactions lead to different movements. If you have an opportunity, interview these individuals after the activity—this will provide you with greater insight into the resulting movement patterns.

7. Finally, design an intervention activity or program that will modify one of the constraints and thereby allow different behaviors to emerge. Focus on things you can do to improve performance for these individuals.

8. You should test this intervention to see if it is feasible. Without testing, you will never really know whether or not the intervention will actually allow new behaviors to emerge!

APPENDIXES

▲▲▲▲▲▲▲▲▲▲▲

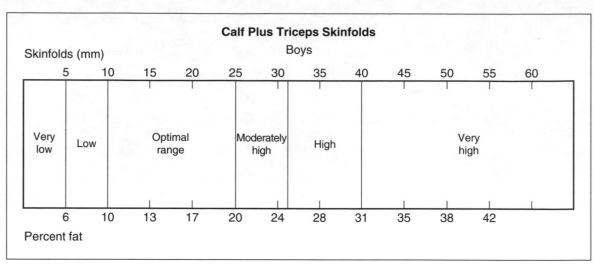

FIGURE A.1

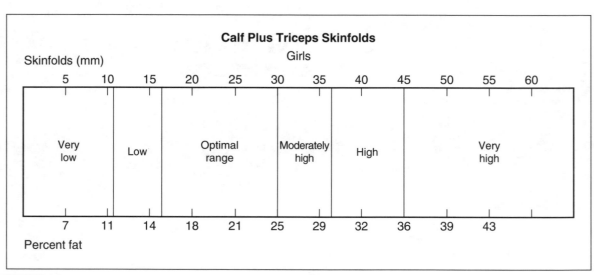

FIGURE A.2

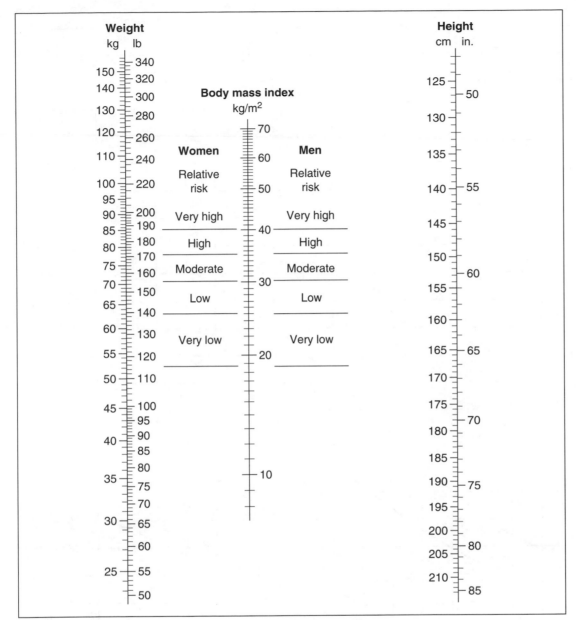

FIGURE B.1 Body mass index chart. Instructions for use: 1) Determine person's height and weight; 2) Connect person's height on chart with person's weight using a ruler or straight edge; 3) Find body mass index at point where ruler or straight edge intersects BMI line; 4) Also, determine appropriate cardiovascular risk from chart (very high, high, moderate, low, very low).

Reprinted, by permission, from G.A. Bray, 1992, "Pathophysiology of obesity," *American Journal of Clinical Nutrition* 55 (2 Suppl), 488S-499S.

TABLE B.1

Interpreting Body Mass Index	
Weight class category	**Body mass index**
Underweight	20
Normal weight	21-24
Overweight	25-29
Obese (very overweight)	30

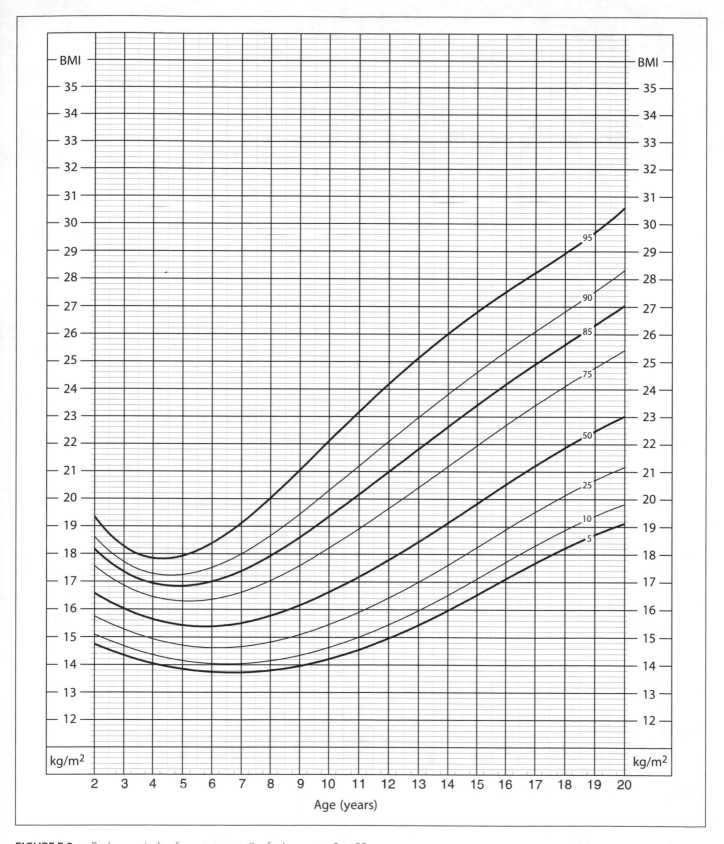

FIGURE B.2a   Body mass index-for-age percentiles for boys, ages 2 to 20 years.

Adapted from **www.cdc.gov/nchs/about/major/nhanes/growthcharts/clinical_charts.htm**. Developed by the National Center for Health Statistics in collaboration with the National Center for Chronic Disease Prevention and Health Promotion (2000).

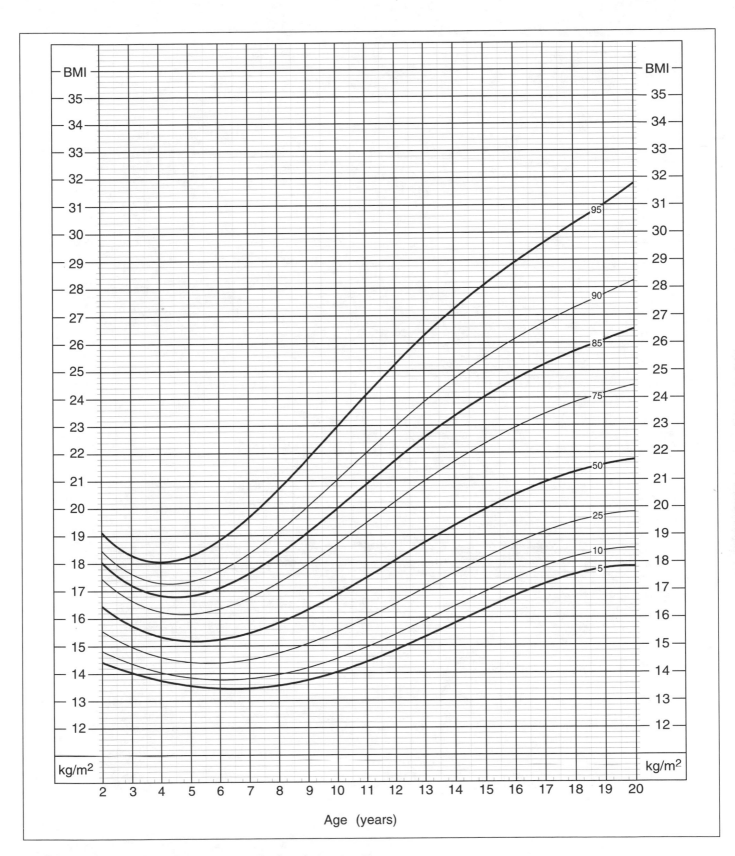

FIGURE B.2b Body mass index-for-age percentiles for girls, ages 2 to 20 years.

Adapted from **www.cdc.gov/nchs/about/major/nhanes/growthcharts/clinical_charts.htm**. Developed by the National Center for Health Statistics in collaboration with the National Center for Chronic Disease Prevention and Health Promotion (2000).

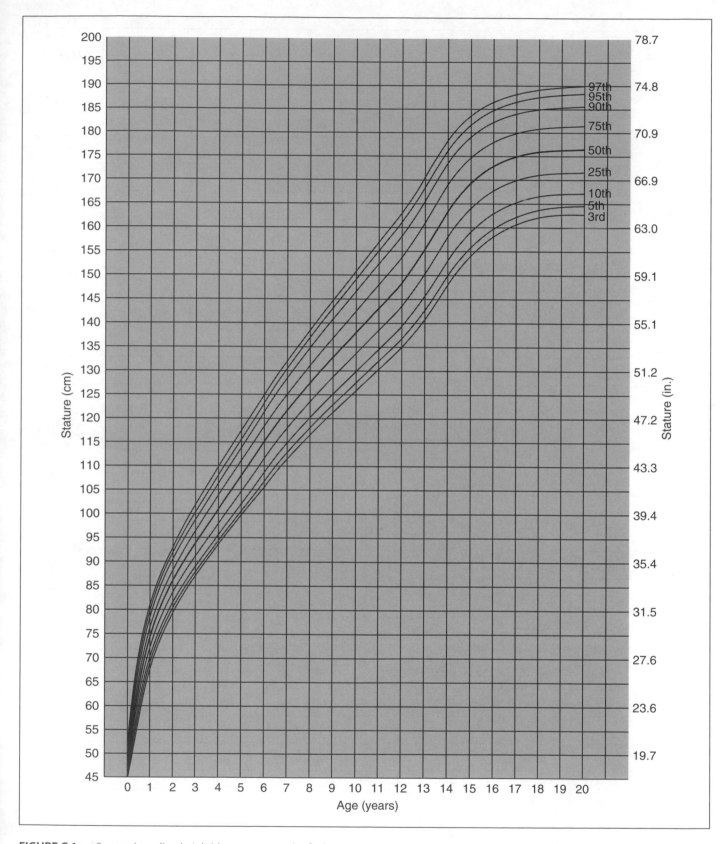

FIGURE C.1a   Stature (standing height) by age percentiles for boys.

Reprinted, by permission, from K.M. Haywood and N. Getchell, 2001, *Life span motor development* (Champaign, IL: Human Kinetics), 49. Adapted from **www.cdc.gov/nchs/about/major/ nhanes/growthcharts/clinical_charts.htm**. Developed by the National Center for Health Statistics in collaboration with the National Center for Chronic Disease Prevention and Health Promotion (2000).

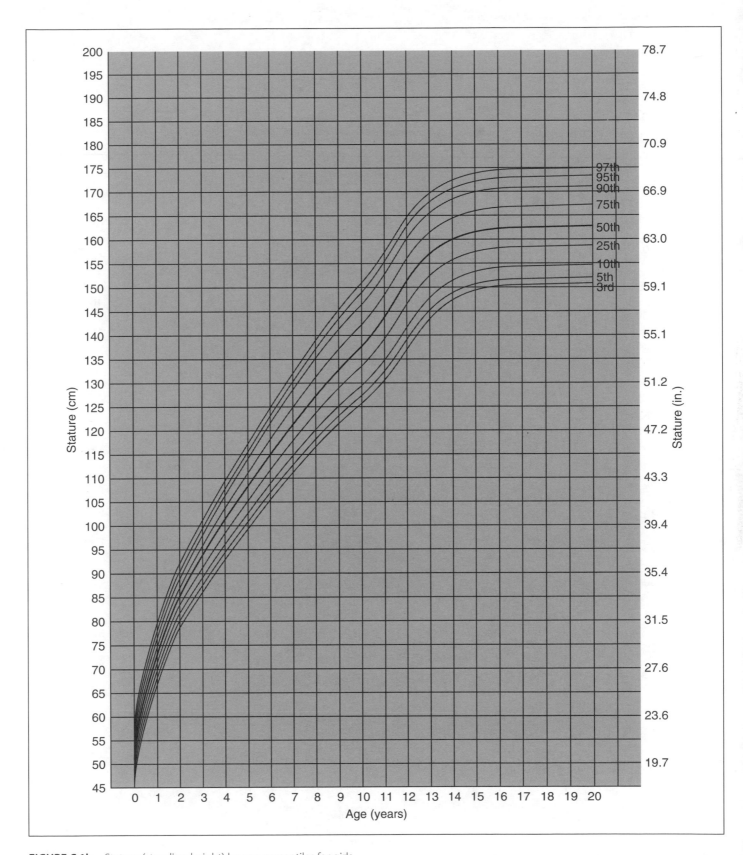

FIGURE C.1b   Stature (standing height) by age percentiles for girls.

Reprinted, by permission, from K.M. Haywood and N. Getchell, 2001, *Life span motor development* (Champaign, IL: Human Kinetics), 50. Adapted from **www.cdc.gov/nchs/about/major/ nhanes/growthcharts/clinical_charts.htm**. Developed by the National Center for Health Statistics in collaboration with the National Center for Chronic Disease Prevention and Health Promotion (2000).

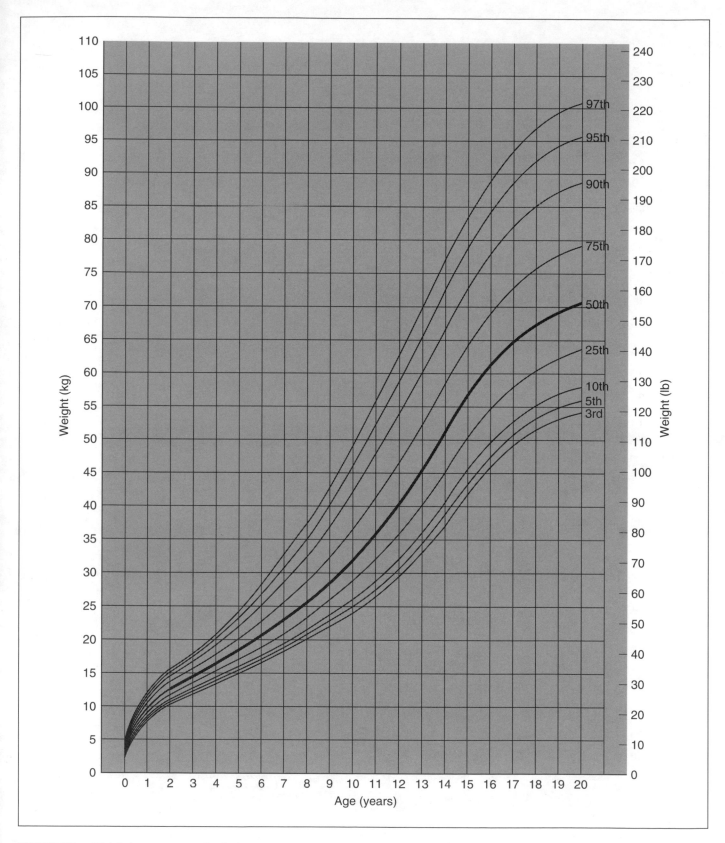

FIGURE C.2a Weight by age percentiles for boys.

Reprinted, by permission, from K.M. Haywood and N. Getchell, 2001, *Life span motor development* (Champaign, IL: Human Kinetics), 51. Adapted from **www.cdc.gov/nchs/about/major/ nhanes/growthcharts/clinical_charts.htm**. Developed by the National Center for Health Statistics in collaboration with the National Center for Chronic Disease Prevention and Health Promotion (2000).

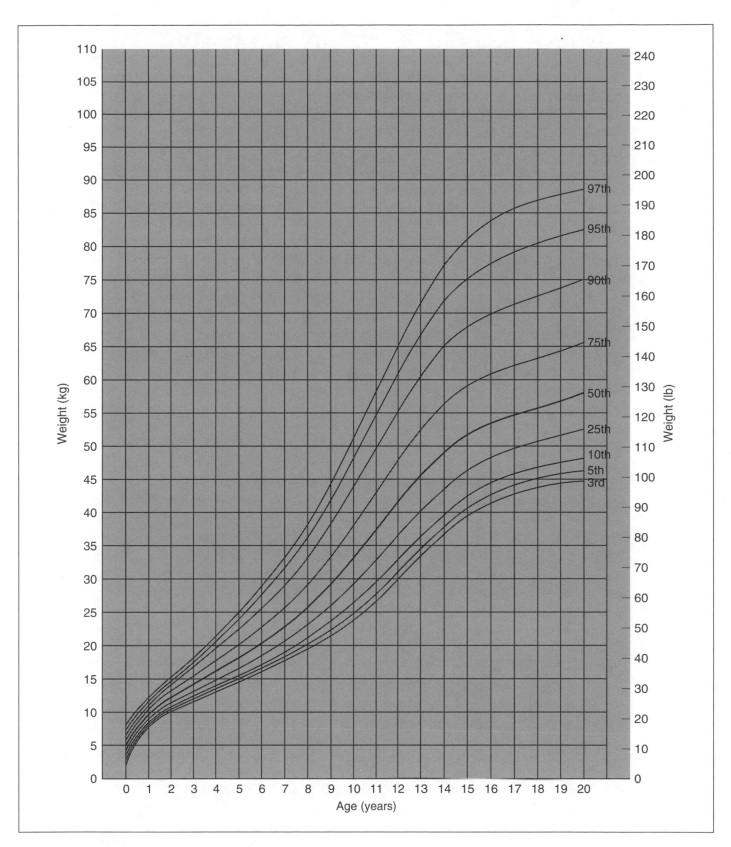

FIGURE C.2b Weight by age percentiles for girls.

Reprinted, by permission, from K.M. Haywood and N. Getchell, 2001, *Life span motor development* (Champaign, IL: Human Kinetics), 52. Adapted from **www.cdc.gov/nchs/about/major/ nhanes/growthcharts/clinical_charts.htm**. Developed by the National Center for Health Statistics in collaboration with the National Center for Chronic Disease Prevention and Health Promotion (2000).

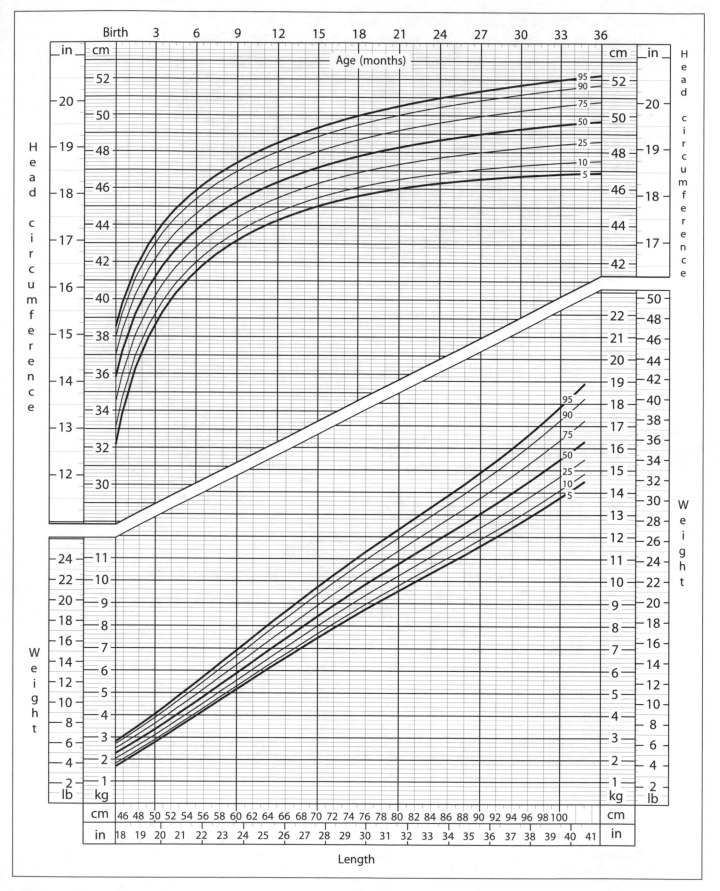

FIGURE D.1a   Head circumference-for-age and weight-for-length percentiles for boys, birth to 36 months.

Reprinted from **www.cdc.gov/nchs/about/major/nhanes/growthcharts/clinical_charts.htm**. Developed by the National Center for Health Statistics in collaboration with the National Center for Chronic Disease Prevention and Health Promotion (2000).

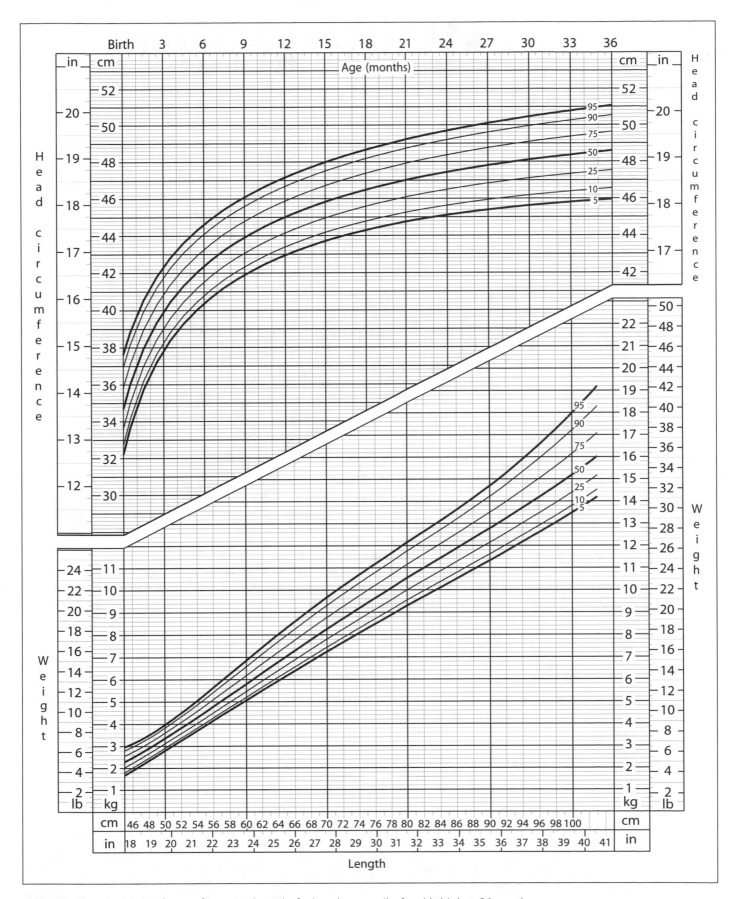

FIGURE D.1b Head circumference-for-age and weight-for-length percentiles for girls, birth to 36 months.

Reprinted from **www.cdc.gov/nchs/about/major/nhanes/growthcharts/clinical_charts.htm**. Developed by the National Center for Health Statistics in collaboration with the National Center for Chronic Disease Prevention and Health Promotion (2000).

Bibliography

Barela, J. A., Jeka, J. J., & Clark, J. E. (1999). The use of somatosensory information during the acquisition of independent upright stance. *Infant Behavior & Development, 22*(1), 87-102.

Bayley, N. (1969). *Manual for the Bayley scales of infant development.* New York: The Psychological Corporation.

Beunen, G., Malina, R. M., Renson, R., & Van Gerven, D. (1988). *Adolescent growth and motor performance: A longitudinal analysis of Belgian boys.* Champaign, IL: Human Kinetics.

Cailliet, R., & Gross, L. (1987). *The rejuvenation strategy.* Garden City, NY: Doubleday.

Clark, E. (1986). *Growing old is not for sissies: Portraits of senior athletes.* Corte Madera, CA: Pomegranate Calendars & Books.

Clark, J. (1994). Motor development. In *Encyclopedia of human behavior.* New York: Academic Press.

Clark, J. E., & Phillips, S.J. (1985). A developmental sequence of the standing long jump. In J. E. Clark & J. H. Humphrey (Eds.), *Motor development: Current selected research* (Vol. 1, pp. 73-85). Princeton, NJ: Princeton Books.

French, K. E., & Thomas, J. R. (1987). The relation of knowledge development to children's basketball performance. *Journal of Sport Psychology, 9,* 15-32.

Gibson, J. J. (1966). *The senses considered as perceptual systems.* Boston: Houghton Mifflin.

Gibson, J. J. (1979). *An ecological approach to visual perception.* Boston: Houghton Mifflin.

Grassi, B., Cerretelli, P., Narici, M. V., & Marconi, C. (1991). Peak anaerobic power in master athletes. *European Journal of Physiology, 62,* 394-399.

Halverson, H. M. (1931). An experimental study of prehension in infants by means of systematic cinema records. *Genetic Psychology Monographs, 10,* 107-286.

Halverson, L. E., Roberton, M. A., & Langendorfer, S. (1982). Development of the overarm throw: Movement and ball velocity changes by seventh grade. *Research Quarterly for Exercise and Sport, 53,* 198-205.

Halverson, L. E., & Williams, K. (1985). Developmental sequences for hopping over distance: A prelongitudinal screening. *Research Quarterly for Exercise and Sport, 56,* 37-44.

Haubenstricker, J. L., Branta, C. F., & Seefeldt, V. D. (1983). *Standards of performance for throwing and catching.* Paper presented at the Annual Conference of the North American Society for Psychology of Sport and Physical Activity, Asilomar, CA.

Jeka, J. J. (1998). Touching surfaces for control, not support. In D. A. Rosenbaum & C. E. Collyer (Eds.), *Timing of behavior: Neural, psychological, and computational perspectives* (pp. 89-105). Cambridge, MA: A Bradford Book, The MIT Press.

Jeka, J. J., & Lackner. J. R. (1994). Fingertip contact influences human postural control. *Experimental Brain Research, 100,* 495-502.

Jeka, J. J., & Lackner. J. R. (1995). The role of haptic cues from rough and slippery surfaces in human postural control. *Experimental Brain Research, 103,* 267-276.

Kasch, F. W., Boyer, J. L., Van Camp, S. P., Verity, L. S., & Wallace, J. P. (1990). The effects of physical activity and inactivity on aerobic power in older men (a longitudinal study). *Physician and Sportsmedicine, 18,* 73-83.

Langendorfer, S. (1980). *Longitudinal evidence for developmental changes in the preparatory phase of the overarm throw for force.* Paper presented at the American Alliance for Health, Physical Education, Recreation and Dance, Detroit, MI.

Langendorfer, S. (1982). *Developmental relationships between throwing and striking: A prelongitudinal test of motor stage theory.* Unpublished doctoral, University of Wisconsin, Madison, WI.

Langendorfer, S. (1990). Motor-task goal as a constraint on developmental status. In J. E. Clark & J. H. Humphrey (Eds.), *Advances in motor development research* (Vol. 3, pp. 16-28). New York: AMS Press.

Langley, D. J., & Knight, S. M. (1996). Exploring practical knowledge: A case study of an experienced senior tennis performer. *Research Quarterly for Exercise and Sport, 67*(4), 433-447.

Leme, S., & Shambes, G. (1978). Immature throwing patterns in normal adult women. *Journal of Human Movement Studies, 4,* 85-93.

McPherson, S. L. (1999). Tactical differences in problem representations and solutions in collegiate varsity and beginner female tennis players. *Research Quarterly for Exercise and Sport, 70*(4), 369-384.

McPherson, S. L., & Thomas, J. R. (1989). Relation of knowledge and performance in boys' tennis: Age and expertise. *Journal of Experimental Child Psychology, 48,* 190-211.

Meredith, M. D., & Welk, G. J. (1999). *FITNESSGRAM test administration manual* (2nd ed.). Champaign, IL: Human Kinetics.

Pyle, S. I. (1971). *A radiographic standard of reference for the growing hand and wrist.* Chicago, IL: Yearbook Medical Publishers.

Reaburn, P. R. J., & Mackinnon, L. T. (1990). Blood lactate response in older swimmers during active and passive recovery following maximal sprint swimming. *European Journal of Applied Physiology, 6,* 246-250.

Roberton, M. A. (1977). Stability of stage categorizations across trials: Implications for the "stage theory" of overarm throw development. *Journal of Human Movement Studies, 3,* 49-59.

Roberton, M. A. (1978a). Longitudinal evidence for developmental stages in the forceful overarm throw. *Journal of Human Movement Studies, 4,* 167-175.

Roberton, M. A. (1983). Changing motor patterns during childhood. In J. R. Thomas (Ed.), *Motor development during childhood and adolescence* (pp. 48-90). Minneapolis: Burgess.

Roberton, M. A. (1984). Changing motor patterns during childhood. In M. V. Ridenour (Ed.), *Motor development: Issues and applications.* Minneapolis: Burgess.

Roberton, M. A. (1988). The weaver's loom: A developmental metaphor. In J. E. Clark & J. H. Humphrey (Eds.), *Advances in motor development research* (Vol. 2, pp. 129-141). New York: AMS Press.

Roberton, M. A., & DiRocco, P. (1981). Validating a motor skill sequence for mentally retarded children. *American Corrective Therapy Journal, 35,* 148-154.

Roberton, M. A., & Halverson, L. E. (1984). *Developing children–Their changing movement.* Philadelphia: Lea & Febiger.

Roberton, M. A., & Langendorfer, S. (1980). Testing motor development sequences across 9-14 years. In D. Nadeau, W. Halliwell, K. Newell, & G. Roberts (Eds.), *Psychology of motor behavior and sport–1979* (pp. 269-279). Champaign, IL: Human Kinetics.

Ross, J. G., Pate, R. R., Delpy, L. A., Gold, R. S., & Svilar, M. (1987). New health-related fitness norms. *Journal of Physical Education, Recreation and Dance, 58,* 66-70.

Seefeldt, V., Reuschlein, S., & Vogel, P. (1972). *Sequencing motor skills within the physical education curriculum.* Paper presented at the American Association for Health, Physical Education, and Recreation, Houston, TX.

Simons, J., Beunen, G. P., Renson, R., Claessens, A. L. M., Vanreusel, B., & Lefevre, J. A. V. (1990). *Growth and fitness of Flemish girls: The Leuven growth study.* Champaign, IL: Human Kinetics.

Spirduso, W. W. (1995). *Physical dimensions of aging.* Champaign, IL: Human Kinetics.

Strohmeyer, H. S., Williams, K., & Schaub-George, D. (1991). Developmental sequences for catching a small ball: A prelongitudinal screening. *Research Quarterly for Exercise and Sport, 62,* 257-266.

Weiner, B. (1974). *Achievement motivation and attribution theory.* Morristown, NJ: General Learning Press.

Weiner, B. (1979). A theory of motivation for some classroom experiences. *Journal of Educational Psychology, 71,* 3-25.

Weiner, B. (1986). *An attributional theory of motivation and emotion.* New York: Springer-Verlag.

Wild, M. (1937). *The behavior pattern of throwing and some observations concerning its course of development in children.* Unpublished Dissertation, University of Wisconsin, Madison.

Williams, K., Haywood, K., & VanSant, A. (1993). Force and accuracy throws by older adult performers. *Journal of Aging and Physical Activity, 1,* 2-12.

Williams, K., Haywood, K., & VanSant, A. (1996). Force and accuracy throws by older adults: II. *Journal of Aging and Physical Activity, 4*(2), 194-202.

About the Authors

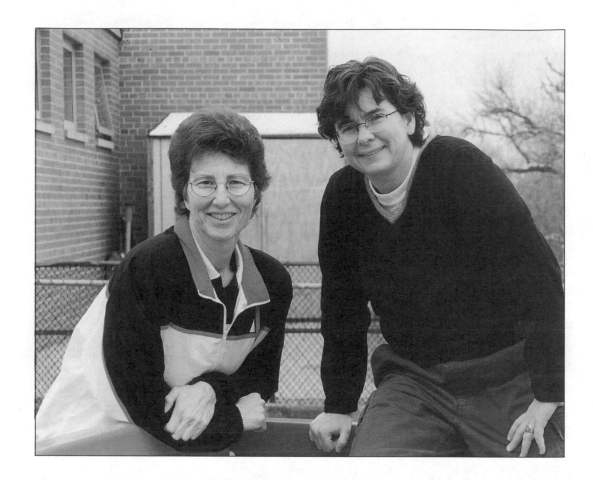

Kathleen M. Haywood, PhD, (left) is associate dean for graduate education at the University of Missouri at St. Louis, where she has taught courses in motor behavior and development, sport psychology, and biomechanics. She has served as secretary/treasurer and president of the North American Society for Psychology of Sport and Physical Activity and as chairperson of the Motor Development Academy of the American Alliance for Health, Physical Education, Recreation and Dance. She also is a recipient of the Alliance's Mabel Lee Award.

Dr. Haywood is also the coauthor of the first and second editions of *Archery: Steps to Success* and *Teaching Archery: Steps to Success.* She earned her PhD in motor behavior from the University of Illinois at Urbana-Champaign in 1976.

Nancy Getchell, PhD, (right) is an assistant professor at the University of Missouri at St. Louis and has been a contributor to the study of motor development for more than 15 years. She is a member of the North American Society for Psychology of Sport and Physical Activity, the International Society of Biomechanics in Sports, and the American Alliance for Health, Physical Education, Recreation and Dance. She is a recipient of the 2001 AAHPERD Lolas E. Halverson Young Investigators Award. She earned a master's degree and PhD in motor development from the University of Wisconsin at Madison.